'Professor Hanson and Professor Green have presented a candid, challenging and thought-provoking response to the question: what makes a person? Their book takes you on a journey through the first 1000 days of life highlighting how physical, environmental and economic factors influence our long-term health. Whether you are a parent already, planning to start a family or simply curious about health, this book will appeal to a wide audience and will most certainly nudge you towards some level of behavioural change.'

Nathan Atkinson, Co-Founder, Rethink Food

'Professor Hanson and Professor Green provide an important view regarding the importance of early fetal development and that as we control our health and exposures we can exert an important influence over the health of our children. They provide the ease of discussion for the lay public, explaining sexual reproduction and the complexities of delivery. They then effectively develop the important concept that long-term health risks like noncommunicable diseases are embedded and the effects impact the next generation. They remind us that the exposures women are subjected to may not be under their control and introduce the concept of "prospective" responsibility – in other words the concept that we all need to work together to ensure that as a society we give the next generation the best start to life.'

Jeanne A. Conry, President, The International Federation of Gynecology and Obstetrics

T0021348

WHAT MAKES A PERSON?

Ever wondered why your life and health can sometimes be so hard to control? Or why it seems so easy for other people? Mark Hanson and Lucy Green draw on their years of experience as scientists and educators to cut through the usual information on genetics and lifestyle to reveal the secrets of early development which start to make each of us unique, during our first 1,000 days from the moment of conception.

Some surprising discoveries, based on little-known new research, show how events during our first 1,000 days make each of us who we are and explain how we control our bodies, processes that go way beyond just the genes which we inherited. Provoking new ways of thinking about being parents, this book empowers individuals and society to give the next generation the gift of a good start to life and future health.

Mark Hanson directs the Institute of Developmental Sciences and is Emeritus British Heart Foundation Professor at the University of Southampton, UK. He is a founder of the International Society for the Developmental Origins of Health and Disease. He is an Honorary Fellow of the Royal College of Obstetricians and Gynaecologists and of the Royal College of Paediatrics and Child Health. He has chaired committees and working groups for the International Federation of Gynecology and Obstetrics, the Partnership for Maternal, Newborn and Child Health and WHO. He researches early developmental environment effects on health across the life course, mechanisms and interventions, in high and low- to middle-income countries. Mark pioneered 'LifeLab' to promote health literacy in school students. He has authored over 400 papers and 11 academic and popular books and advocates application of developmental science to health policy.

Lucy Green researches and teaches early development effects on lifelong health at the University of Southampton. She advocates for the physiological sciences with the International Society for the Developmental Origins of Health and Disease, as a Trustee of the Physiological Society, and as a Fellow of the Royal Society of Biology (where she holds the 2019 Senior Investigator Outreach and Engagement Award), and as Head of Engagement in the Faculty of Medicine. She champions public understanding of science including as a 2018 British Science Association Media Fellow at the BBC, innovating engagement activities for science festivals and devising health-science experiences for young people which enable them to question expert panels and steer the discussion of big health issues. She lives with her family (of 5,000, 6,000 and 20,000 days) in Hampshire.

What Makes a Person?

Secrets of Our First 1,000 Days

MARK HANSON

LUCY GREEN

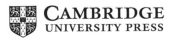

CAMBRIDGE
UNIVERSITY PRESS

CAMBRIDGE
UNIVERSITY PRESS

University Printing House, Cambridge CB2 8BS, United Kingdom

One Liberty Plaza, 20th Floor, New York, NY 10006, USA

477 Williamstown Road, Port Melbourne, VIC 3207, Australia

314–321, 3rd Floor, Plot 3, Splendor Forum, Jasola District Centre, New Delhi – 110025, India

103 Penang Road, #05–06/07, Visioncrest Commercial, Singapore 238467

Cambridge University Press is part of the University of Cambridge.

It furthers the University's mission by disseminating knowledge in the pursuit of education, learning, and research at the highest international levels of excellence.

www.cambridge.org
Information on this title: www.cambridge.org/9781009195256
DOI: 10.1017/9781009195249

First published 2023

Printed in the United Kingdom by TJ Books Limited, Padstow Cornwall

A catalogue record for this publication is available from the British Library.

ISBN 978-1-009-19525-6 Paperback

CONTENTS

FIGURES

PREFACE

Here's a question: do you feel in control of your life?

If you're younger than 16 you'll probably answer 'No' to this question. There are so many things which are uncertain – your next steps towards a career, relationships, where to be … and your actions and decisions tend to be governed by 'grown-ups' and society in general.

If you are in your twenties the answer to the question will probably be 'Yes, I'm in control but …'. You're an adult, but there's lots more to learn and to experience in your life ahead. How much of it will be outside your control is uncertain.

The older you are, the more likely the answer will be 'Yes' – you may be better informed and freer to make decisions about many aspects of life, while also having discovered from experience how many barriers there are and how difficult being 'in control' can be.

Of course, with advancing age, for everyone there comes a time when we feel 'Well, I used to be more in control than I am now'. It seems to be the young and the old who don't feel completely in control of their lives.

Our quality of life is frequently linked to the amount of control we have, or feel that we have, and this in turn is frequently linked to our health – both in terms of how healthy we actually are and how healthy we feel that we are.

There is no doubt that some aspects of our health are within our control. To an extent we can control what we eat, when we get up and when we take exercise. But some things which clearly affect our health are outside our control. Most of us feel that this is particularly true of the genes we have inherited from our parents, over which we had no choice and which we can't control.

Even so, with new technologies and new knowledge about how our genes control our lives come new and grand aspirations that we might be able to engineer the best chance of staying healthy into older age. This might be genetic engineering in the very early embryonic stages of life or personalising medicine to best suit our individual genetic makeup.

This book is about control, but not that kind of control. This is different.

We have written this book to reveal some secrets about a different kind of control that we might have, as parents or as a society, over the first 1,000 days of the lives of the next generation, from conception to the age of two years. It's time that these 'secrets' that are based on major research endeavours around the world over the last 30 years became common knowledge.

This book is about how much we are in control of a particular aspect of our lives – our health. We hope that in reading this book you'll discover that your own ability to be in control, to be healthy for as long as you can, depends on things you may never before have considered.

Before we go on, we should probably ask what being in control means. Whether you are driving a car, planning a party or just walking a dog, there are three parts to it. You need inputs which show how you are doing; you need actions which can change the situation; and you need a control centre to link those actions to the inputs in order to achieve the desired goal – the car stays on the road, the dog stays on the path and the guests, food, drinks and entertainment all come together at the right time and place for the party.

There are aspects of the control of yourself, your body and your health, which you do unconsciously. You don't think about controlling your blood pressure or heart rate, or what goes on in your intestines after you've eaten a meal. You can't control your dreams when you are asleep. But, even without conscious control, these things change with experience, as if we were practising them, influencing them.

Mostly, we think of control over our health in terms of how much we exercise, what we eat, how stressed or tired we are and other aspects of our behaviour or lifestyle. This is of course quite right, and we could add that we learn the importance of these things through experience as well as just being told about them. And we may improve our ability to control our health by practice. In the same way we don't let anyone drive a car alone until they have acquired the necessary skills, both in theory and through practice.

So, going to the gym helps your heart to perform better. Consuming a diet containing enough fibre will improve your digestion and prevent constipation. And watching horror movies late at night is likely to colour your dreams. We have some ability to influence these aspects of our lives. But some people seem naturally to have healthier hearts and guts, and happier dreams than others.

Most of us accept that, however much we teach and practice some things, some people never pass their driving test and some of us really struggle to keep healthy. Then there are some people who seem just 'naturals' at driving a car, a particular sport or living to an old age with good health.

Maybe it's in their genes?

Or maybe not.

Past experience and practice unconsciously changed the ways we control our bodies and our health. This book focusses very specifically on a period of our lives when all this was certainly outside our control

---

This book is about the ways in which past experience and practice unconsciously changed the ways in which we control our bodies and our health. But it focusses very specifically on a period of our lives when all this was most certainly outside our control.

We don't mean the genes you inherited from your parents, over which of course you had no control. We mean the experience and practice that took place at a time when you had no notion of being 'you'. It's the first 1,000 days of your life, from the moment you were conceived until your second birthday.

The clock of your development started to tick then, but you had absolutely no idea about it.

You might feel that exploring your early development is likely to be rather fatalistic and depressing. After all, you can't do anything about what happened during those 1,000 days of your life, all those years ago. If you can't turn the clock back, why bother about it? Wouldn't it be better just to live in the moment, control what you can right now?

No. This book will explain why.

It will show how our first 1,000 days of life was critical for each of us in setting up the control systems in our bodies. Just because you did not consciously choose these control settings for yourself does not mean that they are not highly personal to you and very important.

The first 1,000 days of life is a time about which scientists, doctors, philosophers, as well of course as prospective parents, have thought a great deal. It's probably the time in our lives about which there is more myth, anecdote and superstition than any other. We need to separate the fact from the fiction if we are to understand why this period of our lives matters so much.

We'll see that some seemingly old-fashioned ideas which have been believed for centuries, are proved by recent research to be right. We'll also find that some newer scientific ideas are almost certainly wrong

---

The first 1,000 days is a time in life which is the scene of cutting-edge scientific research and heated debate. A lot of this is not widely known. We'll see that some seemingly old-fashioned ideas about this period of life, which have been believed for centuries, are proved by recent research to be right. We'll also find that some relatively newer scientific ideas are almost certainly wrong.

We'll see that your first 1,000 days of life affects many aspects of your future life. What happened then may even influence how long you will live, how well you live and what is likely to kill you. It isn't just our genes that we pass on to our children. From the moment of conception and for the next 1,000 days we pass on information and signals which will influence how the child's control systems develop.

Of course our developmental processes, by which we become the individuals we all are, don't stop when we are two years old. But research increasingly shows how the stage is set in those first 1,000 days, and how the hidden drama over which we each had no conscious control has been played out. We wrote this book knowing that this is important to how we live and what we do.

To tell the story of our first 1,000 days we could look back and attribute some of our misfortunes to irretrievable problems in our early life, blame our poor genes or our early upbringing. This book does not use this approach.

Instead, we'll suggest that we can use the benefit of hindsight, of knowing the secrets of those 1,000 days, to look forward. Understanding those early days of life could help us understand the ways in which we control our lives more thoroughly and perhaps to make them better in the future. And this may in turn help those who follow us, the next generation, to benefit.

We'll start by looking at what makes the two-year-old the person they are, with their unique personality and very definite place in the world. They are now in control of their lives in some ways, although definitely not in others. We won't be providing a manual on how to bring up a baby or infant – there are many of those already. For the parents of a toddler reading this, we hope to provide insights and new ways of thinking about child development, but not advice.

In Chapter 2 we'll go back to the beginning of our childhood, to birth itself, to ask questions about what happens during this risky time in our lives. Birth is dangerous – some experts would say that, after the danger of our final moments on this planet, being born comes second in terms of life-threatening risk. Who's in control then?

Chapter 3 will take us back into the womb, to explore the amazing life of the unborn baby, or fetus. This isn't a textbook for medical students, nurses or midwives – there are many such books already. But exciting new scientific discoveries mean that the mysteries of pregnancy have got fewer. At a time when no-one is watching, fetal organs and control systems are developing, and so are aspects of behaviour too. The pattern of this development of the fetus is of huge importance for lifelong health.

Going back from fetal life we arrive in Chapter 4 at conception – sex. You might think that there wouldn't be anything very interesting to consider in the development of a simple little embryo before it becomes a fetus at about 50–60 days into its first 1,000 days. You would be wrong. New discoveries have shown just how important this time in our lives was, and is.

The inequalities and inequities which already existed have been dramatically widened and worsened by the COVID-19 pandemic everywhere

---

Chapter 5 gives us the opportunity to think more globally, about how the events leading up to the first 1,000 days affect our health as adults, and the implications for equity and social justice across genders, social groups and ethnicities. These have enormous importance for society, and not just for girls and women or for mothers, and the tendency to put the blame on them is something which we strongly denounce. The inequalities and inequities which already existed have been dramatically widened and worsened by the COVID-19 pandemic everywhere.

The last chapter in this book will ask what we all can do to make the lives of the next generation as good as possible. Now that we know some of the secrets of our lives in the first 1,000 days, how can we pass on the best gift ever, of a good start at that time, to the next generation?

We felt that this story is best told by starting at the end and working back, like the detective arriving on the crime scene who traces back the clues they uncover to discover what happened. Our first 1,000 days led up to the age of two. So that will be the start of the story.

1 NOW YOU ARE TWO: THE END OF THE BEGINNING?

Memories Are Made of This

How much do you remember about your life before your second birthday, during your infancy? Where you lived, your brothers and sisters, how your parents or the people who cared for you behaved, being breast- or bottle-fed and your first weaning foods?

Almost certainly, if you're honest, the answer to this question will be 'I can't remember any of it'.

But you might know people who have memories of a time when they were one year old, seeing someone from their baby cot or sitting in a high chair, perhaps tipping food onto the floor.

Most families love storytelling, and events in our early lives can easily become mythologised to seem as vivid in our minds as those experiences we had when we were older and consciously witnessed them. So while you might think that you have a memory of events in those first two years, on closer examination it usually turns out to be imagined, based on later experiences or what was told to you by people who were older. After all, it's quite likely that your family lived in the same home for more than just your first two years and even more likely that you had the same brothers and sisters and carers.

It's a natural human tendency to make connections between the past and the present and there are traditions in many cultures about this. They range from giving a child a name from a previous generation, to more complex beliefs, for example that the souls of ancestors live in hollow stones after their death until they are able to emerge to inhabit the bodies of children.

But *why* don't we remember anything about these formative two years of our lives?

Despite considerable research on how our minds work, the fact is that we don't know the answer to this question.

Later in our lives we can (usually) remember the first time that we met someone, especially if they turned out to be significant to us in some way. We can remember how, on that first occasion, we saw them and interacted with them as a new person, someone different from the people we'd met before.

But how did we know that they were new to us? That requires experience. Could it be that without having met lots of different people we can't say whether or not someone we meet is new to us?

Maybe what we call memories can't really occur until we are old enough to have built up a stock of experience on which to base new events or encounters. Memories require a system for categorising experience, for cataloguing it and filing it under headings that allow it to be retrieved later.

Without experience of what it is like to be a grown-up human being, how does the child grow up to be just that, a grown-up human being?

Without any experience or prior knowledge of what it is like to be a grown-up human being, how does the child manage to grow up to be just that, a grown-up human being?

It's a shame we can't remember events in those first 1,000 days because so much was happening to us then. We took our first steps, literally as well as metaphorically, in a challenging but stimulating new world.

The first two years of infancy are recognised by health professionals as being a critical phase in our development. So we need to delve deeper into them if we are to understand what makes each of us.

You Get That from Your Father

It's a source of delight, or perhaps sometimes of dismay, for parents to see some of their best, or possibly their worst, features reflected in their offspring. Why do some characteristics, from the length of noses to the ability to sing in tune, get passed from one generation to the next, while others do not? Is it largely a question of chance or the accident of development? How much is Nature and how much is Nurture? This an age-old question which has been debated many, many times and from different standpoints – social, emotional, religious, legal as well as scientific to name only a few. The balance of opinion has swung back and forth over the years as new evidence appeared and particular views gained prominence.

For many years the most widely accepted view has been that 'nature', our inborn characteristics which are hard to change, is driven by the genes which we inherited. Identifying and mapping all our genes was the amazing achievement of the Human Genome Project at the start of this millennium. Knowing this sequence seemed to hold most if not all of the answers to questions about human nature, including how the tiny embryo grows into a baby and why we differ as individuals. It was a little surprising that it turned out that we possess only 20,000–25,000 genes. Are these enough to make something as complicated as a person? In addition, it turned out that we share 99% of our genes with our nearest cousins, the chimpanzees. About

50% of our genes are the same as bananas. This made us realise that what our genes are – their nature and their sequence in the DNA strand – was only part of the story. Equally, or perhaps even more importantly, might be how those genes are used and the process which controls how they work during the development of a person, a chimp or a banana.

About 50% of our genes are the same as bananas

This challenge took us back to basics. At the end of the nineteenth century a monk named Gregor Mendel worked out the mathematics of inheritance from a series of breeding experiments using peas. He calculated rules by which certain characteristics are passed from one generation to the next by looking at the offspring of peas, with certain characteristics such as colour and skin texture, which he had cross-pollinated. Even though he had no idea of the existence of DNA, let alone the genes it makes up, it turned out that these characteristics are inherited in a strictly mathematical way, so that the likelihood of an individual pea plant having a particular characteristic could be calculated with certainty from the characteristics of its parent plants. Random effects, or effects of the weather had no influence on this inheritance.

These rules of so-called Mendelian inheritance apply to a few of our characteristics such as the colour of our eyes, and to some diseases which run in families such as cystic fibrosis. It is possible to predict the chance that a child will inherit these characteristics if we know the genetic make-up of the parents, just as Mendel was able to do with his breeding experiments in peas.

But most of our physical characteristics don't follow Mendel's rules. They may depend on the inheritance of a large number of genes, which interact to produce a characteristic and can be inherited in various combinations. The dependence on such a large number might give the appearance of a more random inheritance, and would have defeated Mendel's mathematics and his experimental design. Today we can explore such inheritance through our ability to define the nature of thousands of genes from an individual and having the software to look for patterns. But there is also another possibility which could explain why some of the variation in characteristics between members of a family do not appear to follow Mendel's rules. Other non-genetic factors during very early life, such as exposure to hormones or nutrients, can influence whether the inherited genes actually work in a way that leads to a characteristic being developed in the unborn baby. The tiny 'epigenetic' marks left on DNA alter the way cells in our bodies make vital proteins, and so our characteristics, and we talk more about them in Chapter 5.

Despite expectations, the publication of the Human Genome hasn't led to the identification of a strongly genetic basis for the explained inheritance of many of our characteristics. Nor has it explained the basis for risk of the chronic diseases which account for the majority of deaths worldwide every year, even though there is plenty of evidence that these diseases can be passed from one generation to the next.

And it's not just physical. Finding a purely genetic basis for inheritance becomes even more problematic with more complex characteristics like aspects of behaviour, such as aggression. It is complex because behaviour is the result of lots of parts of the brain working in conjunction with the rest of the body. Even in a 'simple' organism such as the fruit fly, which has about 10,000 fewer genes than we do, aggressive behaviour results from the action of numerous genes.

An often-quoted example of genetic influences concerns the differences in behaviours between boys and girls. After all, the sexes are genetically different, at least in terms of girls having two X chromosomes and boys one X and one Y chromosome. So how much of the behavioural differences between boys and girls is genetic, and how much is due to environmental factors?

This question has occupied child psychologists, researchers and those concerned with gender issues as well as, of course, billions of parents, for generations.

It is clear that a preference for dolls and pink clothes is not a genetic predisposition in girls. The preferences of our children and many of their behaviours are down to the encouragement they receive from the obvious delight in their parents or carers when they choose certain things, and the discouragement for other things. Don't forget that in the 1920s pink was still a 'boy's colour'.

One morning the boy had chewed his toast into the shape of a handgun and was shooting at his sister across the breakfast table

---

But of course it isn't just parents and carers – all sorts of other influences operate. We can only sympathise with the young parents who were determined that their little boy would not become an aggressive young lad like so many older children in the town where they lived. They were adamant that he would not see violence on TV, would have no toy soldiers and certainly no plastic swords or cannons. But kids will use their imagination to create their own games. Imagine their dismay when one morning the boy had chewed his toast into the shape of a handgun and was shooting at his sister across the breakfast table.

Born Losers

The Nature versus Nurture distinction becomes really dangerous, and unethical, when it is used for social engineering or to argue for the maintenance of the status quo. The issue is encapsulated by the views of the psychologist Francis Galton who coined the terms Nature and Nurture in 1869.

Galton was a firm believer in the values of mid-Victorian society in Britain – where there was a place for everyone and everyone should stay in their place. The importance of inheritance of each place in society meant that breeding needed to be controlled in what were seen to be the lower social classes to prevent their numbers getting out of hand.

So Galton was the father of the eugenics movement. His book *Hereditary Genius* celebrated the most influential families of his time, where he argued that children would prosper and gain acclaim because they had inherited the necessary talents from their parents. The uneducated, the poor and the feckless would achieve little because they had not inherited these attributes from their parents, and nor could they pass them on to their children. So social mobility was limited by this self-fulfilling prophesy. Galton saw such 'innate' differences as part of Nature. They could not be modified very much by childhood environment and upbringing, in other words by Nurture.

Disagreeable though it is, Galton's distinction between Nature and Nurture is still with us to an extent even today. Some researchers still maintain, based for example on following up the achievements of adopted children compared to those brought up by their biological parents, that the environment of the family home, and even the quality of education at school, plays a lesser part than inherited genetic characteristics in determining a child's future. Ideas like this – that who we are is largely based on the genes that we inherited – can even lead to believing that some members of society should not be allowed to conceive a child.

These sorts of societal judgements can have horrifying consequences, for example the 'rescue' of children of unmarried Catholic mothers in Ireland. These girls and women were judged unfit to be mothers even if for reasons of circumstance rather than genetics. Poor care of their children led to many fatalities and their forced adoption to enormous and lifelong trauma. Some of these homes for unmarried mothers and their children were not closed until the 1990s.

Later in this book we'll explain the new scientific reasons for why a hard distinction between Nature and Nurture is biologically incorrect as well as socially dangerous. For now we might remember that nearly a century before Galton, in 1776, Thomas Jefferson wrote in the US Declaration of Independence: 'All men are created equal', sowing the seeds for the human rights movement:

> ... all men are created equal, that they are endowed by their Creator with certain unalienable Rights, that among these are Life, Liberty and the Pursuit of Happiness.
>
> Thomas Jefferson, US Declaration of Independence in 1776

For us the key to this declaration is that every child should have the opportunity, or in other words be 'nurtured', to fulfil their potential irrespective of their parents and what they may have inherited from them by 'Nature'. Ignoring this principle leads to inequity and social injustice. The word 'created' would have had religious implications in Thomas Jefferson's day. But the 'unalienable Rights' with which we are all 'endowed', we now believe, would include a healthy first 1,000 days, and a supportive society which ensures fairness regardless of how we develop. We'll come back to these ideas later.

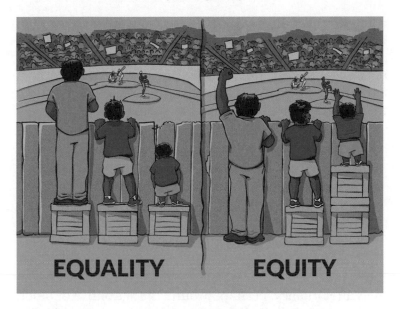

Figure 1.1 Equality or equity? Every child deserves the opportunity to fulfil their potential irrespective of their parents and what they may have inherited from them by 'Nature'. To be fair or equitable, this does not mean giving every child the same, and might require some redistribution of resources.
Interaction Institute for Social Change. Artist: Angus Maguire.

Who Cares for You?

To take the story further, we must think about how the child interacts with the environment and their carers. How much can they really change the child's development?

We can get some idea of just how much from children brought up in extreme or very unusual conditions. Take for example the stories in folklore about children who were reared by animals. The most famous is Mowgli in Rudyard Kipling's *The Jungle Book*, published in 1907. In the story, Mowgli is lost in the jungle in India after his parents are attacked by a tiger and is then brought up by wolf parents. He develops great skill as a hunter and tracker and when he eventually returns to human society he becomes a jungle ranger. He is very different from other young men but his time with the wolves had not prevented his development of many human characteristics. The popularity of the first Mowgli story led Kipling to write many others about him. They are imaginative, if far-fetched, but, like many of the best stories, they have some basis in reality.

There are documented cases of children being reared by animals, from monkeys to dogs, bears and goats. In some, a baby only a few months old is adopted by furry parents

---

There are in fact quite a few documented cases of children being reared by animals, from monkeys to dogs, bears and goats. In most, the child is left to live with animals after infancy, perhaps around the age of five or older. But in some a baby only a few months old is adopted by its new furry parents. The results seem similar though. When the child is discovered some years later, they are unable to speak, prefer to run around on all fours and have little interest or understanding of human social norms. So distinctly non-human behaviours can develop in a child, for example being wolf-like, without having inherited wolf genes. Unlike Mowgli in Kipling's story though, these children were not easily socialised and had what we would describe as severe behavioural disorders.

Clearer lessons about the importance of our early environment can be learned from children who have been exposed from birth to institutional life in which they were neglected or abused. Some of the most harrowing accounts come from the Romanian 'orphanages'.

In 1966 the hard-line dictator Ceauşescu decreed that contraception and abortion were illegal in Romania, supposedly in an attempt to prevent the country's population falling even more after the effects of the Second World War in reducing it. Abortion was only permitted if the woman was over 40 or already had four children. Even rape was not considered to be a sufficient reason for the termination of pregnancy. To enforce compliance with Ceauşescu's unethical plan even further, in 1977 taxation was levied on people who remained childless. As a result, many children were abandoned in so-called orphanages, often because their mothers or parents could not afford to keep them. This became especially true after 1982 when the country's economic situation deteriorated even further. Overall, there may have been as many as half a million children institutionalised.

The conditions in the orphanages were terrible, with little heating or food and low levels of poorly paid, untrained staff who often showed no care for or even abused their little charges. Children were sometimes confined together in cots for days in unsanitary conditions. Needless to say, the emotional damage to these 'orphans' was extreme and both their physical and mental development was delayed. For example, their language skills were very poor.

After the fall of Ceauşescu's regime in the revolution of 1989, conditions in Romania were initially even worse for a time. But by the 1990s and early 2000s programmes to adopt some of the Romanian children to homes overseas were underway. Not all these adoptees went to good homes, unfortunately, but those who were lucky were usually able to catch up in terms of language and mental development.

The ability to catch up was greater in those children adopted before the age of two – the end of their first 1,000 days – than in children adopted at an older age. Research has shown that this was not because the younger children had been exposed to a shorter period of abuse, although this of course would be true, but because rescuing them before their first 1,000 days were over gave greater opportunities to get their development back on track, to learn new skills such as language. It's much easier to influence our development during the period when it's still very plastic.

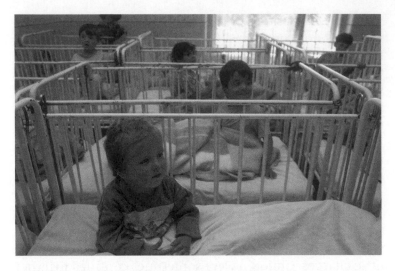

Figure 1.2 Children in an orphanage in Romania The conditions and disruption to young children's lives affected both their physical and mental development.
BSIP/Universal Images Group/Getty Images.

Just as with a plastic spoon, plasticity has limits. Bend it a little and the spoon may return to its original shape; bend it some more and it may break or stay bent

This idea of plasticity – the potential to change and to develop in different ways – has been probably understood since the beginning of time, even if it wasn't formally recorded. But just as with an object such as a spoon which is made of plastic, plasticity has limits. Bend it a little and the spoon may return to its original shape; bend it some more and it may break or stay bent. Our plasticity during development is limited in a similar way, because an extreme stress may be just too damaging to allow recovery. But there is another aspect which is at least as important, and this is that developmental plasticity is time-limited.

Once the period during which it is possible to change and adapt has passed, the opportunity to be plastic is no longer there. So preventing children from experiencing severe deprivation before the first 1,000 days is key to avoiding more damaging and irreversible consequences. This was something which we can learn from the horrors of the Romanian orphanages.

Making up later for a poor start to life can be very difficult. Anyone who has managed to achieve what is called social mobility – the achievement of better socio-economic position even after a poor start to life – will know this very well. We are reminded of the work of Frederick Douglass, born into slavery on a plantation in Maryland in about 1818. After he managed to escape many years later, he became actively involved in writing and speaking out about the evils of slavery and the case for its abolition. In 1855 he wrote: 'It is easier to build strong children than to mend broken men'. This is something that politicians and those who exercise power everywhere should remember. Whether through education or other measures to assist disadvantaged members of the population, investment in early life may not be easy, but the consequences of not doing so are even more difficult to fix.

Parrot Fashion

One of the things which is clear from the Mowgli stories and the horrifying experiences of the Romanian orphans is that the development of language is very plastic. Perhaps this is because it is such a powerful tool, so getting it right really matters.

Once the young child starts to speak, they quickly seem to realise this power. They attract the attention of adults and engage them in all sorts of new ways, sometimes making it easier to influence those grown-ups to provide what the child wants.

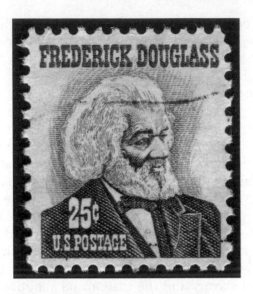

Figure 1.3 Frederick Douglass (1818–1895)
A powerful campaigner for the abolition
of slavery, based on his own personal
experience.
Traveler1116/Getty Images.

Some children seem to go through a difficult phase, with temper tantrums which are a cause of concern to their parents, before they acquire much in the way of speech, as if they are rather frustrated with their inability to communicate. But from around 18 months of age, the child seems to pick up and use new words on a daily basis. This will be well-received by parents or carers – after all it's much easier to get along with someone who can explain their needs and feelings in words – and so this reinforces learning mechanisms which work fast to memorise and retrieve useful words.

Parents are naturally delighted to hear their child's first word or phrase. Will it be 'computer' or 'picture'? Will it be a word that has been linked to an action like 'clap'?

Or will it be an embarrassing word picked up by hearing something they shouldn't have heard, in parrot fashion? In truth the child's first word is likely not to have a great deal of significance in the long term and will soon be followed by others with different connotations. All children will try out new words at first, to see if they get the expected reaction and were the right ones to say. It takes practice. This emphasises just how important it is to talk to children from an early age, even though they may not seem to understand and certainly won't reply. They take on board much more than we realise and store the information away for future use.

Is language acquisition a specifically human characteristic? Perhaps it is, because although many other species have the ability to communicate by making sounds in various ways, from woodpeckers pecking to the high frequency calls of bats and the low frequency calls of whales, only the unique structure of the human mouth, tongue and voicebox or larynx allows our complex language communication. But that alone does not explain how, at a certain age, a child starts to speak to their parents in a language which they understand – Spanish, Cantonese, Finnish, whatever. Nor does the genetic basis for the structure and function of the human larynx explain how we partly acquire language from seeing written words as well as hearing them and trying to pronounce them.

The usefulness of language acquisition, even the need for language perhaps, could be genetically encoded and inherited by us all in a reliable way, but the process and the end result are clearly different. So the child growing up in a Greek-speaking family does not start to speak Dutch.

Learning on the Job

We learn much of how to behave as humans on the job, so to speak.

The key here is the word 'learn'. This is an aspect of our development which we see easily but, unlike our purely genetic inherited characteristics, there is no simple explanation of the process of learning. It must be sufficiently complex to accommodate all the possibilities of human experience and behaviour – maybe growing up in the arctic and learning how to survive the winter by catching fish through holes in the ice, or how safely you can cross a busy city street.

The possibilities are endless, but we only keep those behaviours and ideas that we learn are important, at least to the person we are becoming and the world in which we find ourselves.

We all experience sometimes the sensation of being overwhelmed with information. On a good day, we can summon up skills we've learned to deal with this overload, to filter the information, prioritise what we will pay attention to and incorporate this into our actions. But imagine the brain of a young child. Through their eyes, ears and sense of touch, taste and smell, millions of items of information about the world are being sent to their brain every second. They can't all be stored or even processed.

How does the young child make sense of it all? How can they decide what matters?

The challenge is made even more acute because time is limited, so the young child has to be a quick learner. As many as 50% of the neurons in the baby's brain at birth have shrunk to be inoperative by the time that they become adult. This process is fastest in the young child but is probably not complete until early adulthood. The neurons shrink because they did not make helpful, or much-used, connections. In addition, the neurons that remain – and there are still about 86 billion of them – have pruned down the number of connections which they make with each other, selecting only those that they use.

When you set up a new mobile phone you know that you could connect it to any of the 3.5 billion other phone users in the world. Your phone is potentially connected to all of them. But you decide to store only a tiny fraction of these potential phone numbers, perhaps a hundred at the most, in your contacts list. These belong to the people whom you regularly contact or need to access easily. So you have made a choice about which numbers to store.

In just the same way, the developing brain 'chooses' to keep the connections between neurons which are operative and useful, and to delete the rest. The key is that those neurons which talk to one another through their nerve fibres and tiny connections (called synapses) stay connected.

In addition, the neurons 'talk' to one another based on experience. In our infancy we very quickly learn to recognise the faces and the voices of the people whom we see most often and who are most significant to us, usually our parents or carers and our siblings. As these people are felt to be important, the neurons processing this information will get good at talking to each other to allow rapid recognition of these faces and voices.

Tuning of the connections in our brains, based on experience, depends on how common a particular experience is, such as how often we see a particular face or hear a particular voice

---

So the tuning of the connections in our brains, based on experience, depends on how common a particular experience is, such as how often we see a particular face or hear a particular voice. It will also depend on how powerful a stimulus is, for example the strong feeling of contentment when someone feeds us if we are hungry. Equally, a very frightening or painful experience is likely to preserve the neuronal circuitry we used to experience it, even if it only occurred once. Even a young child who touches a very hot stove is unlikely to do so again.

All this tuning of the neurons in our brains – the developmental plasticity we noted earlier– goes on automatically in each of us. It does not involve any conscious control, at least by the young 'self'.

Many of the components of our bodies can be fine-tuned like this during their development, according to what we are experiencing. It might be refining the number of individual cells that make up an organ or the functional control settings of these cells.

We'll all have different experiences in our early lives and so developmental plasticity provides lots of room for individuality. We all grow differently and grow up to be individuals. Some of this development we see played out before our eyes, like behaviour, and some happens out of sight inside our bodies, such as how many muscle cells we develop in our hearts, as we'll discuss later.

We often think of this individuality in terms of the 'personality' which a child develops. This is clearly a gradual process, and in many ways it may not be finalised until the complete maturation of the so-called higher executive functions of the brain which control decision-making, a sense of responsibility etc. New brain imaging techniques have shown that this isn't complete until we are in our late twenties. Perhaps only then is personality finally set in our lives – or perhaps it's never set. But much of what makes each of us a unique person takes place over our first 1,000 days.

Even young babies show differences in personality, for example in their responses to a new stimulus or experience. Some find a new object or a new face interesting, others find it disturbing, and still others seem to treat it with equanimity. These different responses will, in time, evoke a range of reactions from adults, which in turn may inhibit or enhance them in the child, and so the process of developing into a unique individual goes on.

This is all part of the learning process, and again emphasises the importance of stimulating and interacting with the child in a reassuring way in order to reinforce reciprocal interaction and socialisation. We evolved to be a highly social species, and the sooner we learn the importance of social skills the better. Many parents find that young children will become demanding just at the time that they start browsing social media on their phone, or settle to watch a favourite TV programme. The child soon detects that the adult isn't paying attention to them and attempts to change the situation. In addition, new research using monitoring of brain function is revealing that young children who spend several hours a day on screen-based activities – whether on a computer or watching TV – show altered executive functions which are likely to make them find it hard to focus and concentrate on tasks when they later attend school. This is a rapidly moving field of research and is likely to have important implications for childcare.

A mother of a two-year-old was puzzled that he seemed to wave his hand back and forth whenever she reprimanded him for naughtiness, that is, until she realised this was what he had learned to do on an iPad in order to change what he saw

---

What the child learns early isn't necessarily what parents or carers, or indeed society in general, will see as acceptable social behaviour. A mother of a two-year-old was puzzled that he seemed to wave his hand back and forth whenever she reprimanded him for naughtiness, that is, until she realised this was what he had learned to do on an iPad in order to change what he saw – if she seems cross just swipe her away!

Tickling the Senses

For a child to learn things about the world there are some basics that need to be in place. These include structural components of the body. Making them is in essence driven by the genes we inherit from our parents. Then comes the process of checking the way that these basics are working against rules laid down in the society and environment where we live, and against our past experiences. This learning process applies across all our body's cells, organs and systems. Having rules makes such learning less complicated than it might seem.

One visual shortcut is in detecting edges and outlines of objects, and this may also explain the odd fear that cats have of cucumbers – a case of mistaken identity based on a snake-like outline perhaps?

Take for example sight – our visual system. The visual system is extraordinary in its precision. But it also has useful shortcuts to save time and simplify the visual processing required. One way is in detecting edges and the outlines of objects, helpful for example for speedy recognition of a symbol on a road sign while driving. Maybe it also explains the odd fear that cats have of cucumbers – a case of mistaken identity based on a snake-like outline perhaps?

Detecting movement is another shortcut our visual system uses to speed up the detection of critical aspects of the visual world. Many animals are much better at this than we are, especially predators like cats. But even in the young child, the processing of sensory information by the brain must be very clever if the child is to make sense of their world. Imagine the child sitting comfortably in their chair when their brain detects that a favourite soft toy is moving. This is a surprise, but something is happening because the toy is moving across the child's visual field.

Now the brain has to decide whether the toy is actually moving. Maybe it just appears to be moving because the child's eyes have moved, or their head has swivelled or their body has shifted sideways. We can scarcely imagine the complexity of the brain's software which allows it to use all the inputs from the retina, the muscles attached to the eyeball and those in the neck and body, to decide what has happened and which of these possibilities is correct. Within much less than a second the child's brain has figured all this out, and the child shows surprise or delight, or simply ignores the information.

Some fundamental anatomical properties of our eyes are basically fixed and can't be changed. But the visual system takes a while to develop its full function and, while it's developing, it's learning from experience, rather like machine-learning in a computer artificial intelligence program. In some experiments in psychology many years ago, researchers raised kittens in environments which featured predominantly horizontal or vertical lines. When the cats were adult, their visual systems were found to respond largely to images containing either horizontal or vertical lines.

Although it takes some time for the lens of the baby's eye to take up the appropriate shape in order to focus on objects, it can initially see those which are fairly close to the face. The rod receptors in the retina which detect levels of light, and the three types of cone receptors which detect ranges of colours in our visual range, are functional at birth.

The nerve fibres from the retina which send visual information to the processing neurons in the brain are there too. They will eventually connect to columns of cells in the outer layers of the brain to make a map of the visual world, rather like the pixels of a digital camera image. The process of making these cell columns takes time and is based on experience over that time. Once formed, their connections and the aspects of the visual world to which they respond cannot be altered.

Animals differ in the extent to which their visual processing systems are developed at birth. The newborn lamb obviously has a much more mature processing capability than the human infant. Unlike many other newborn animals which can take time to develop in the safety of the nest, the lamb quickly has to fend for itself. Not only can the lamb walk around within a few minutes of being born, even if rather wobbly, but it has to find its own way to the mother's teat which will supply its first meal. It can soon navigate obstacles such as rocks or trees and even has a good three-dimensional sense of depth, which will be useful if it's been born on a steep hillside.

We humans are way behind this at birth. Very similar processes to vision operate for the baby's other sensory systems – hearing, smell, taste and touch. All these senses feed into a map on the surface of the brain with an area of the map to do with vision, and areas for the other senses. For the skin, the receptors for light touch, deep pressure, heat, cold and pain for large areas of the body feed into parts of the mapping area. In the newborn baby the map is diffuse and not well focussed. With experience and time, the mapping becomes more accurate and detailed.

In early life the baby may not be able to discriminate between stimuli such as touch, pain, hot and cold over much of the arms or legs. As the focussing proceeds however, the discrimination becomes much finer, extending down to the fingers and toes until eventually the very accurate sensory perception we have, especially in our fingers, is achieved. This is made possible by the much greater number of sensory receptors in the skin of our fingers than, say, our backs. So the size of the area of the brain associated with sensory perception in the different parts of our body depends on the number of receptors and their importance in our lives. The face, and particularly the lips, has large representation, as do the fingers and toes, while the torso has much less.

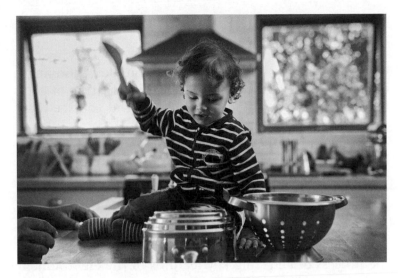

Figure 1.4 Exploring the world around us The development of the child's responses to the world critically depends on interaction with their environment – testing the limits of things in their path, sensing with their whole body. This is happening in plain sight after birth. But it does not require expensive toys or games. It's the everyday world they need to explore.
Dean Mitchell/Getty Images.

We've now arrived at a really important point in our story, which is that the development of the child's responses to the world critically depends on interaction with the environment. And this makes the possibilities for individuality endless. Making a person is a lot more varied and interesting than genes and inherited 'nature'.

Just Checking

One of the essential aspects of the child's development, as with any learning process, is checking. If you're learning a language, and your teacher uses a new word which you haven't heard before, you will try to repeat it and check that your pronunciation is good enough and that you're using it in the right context.

Watch a child who is doing something that they are fairly sure is naughty – they may look around questioningly to check the response they get. The same is true of good behaviour – it's as if they're thinking 'Did you see that? Aren't I good ... Where's my reward?'

This sounds rather as if the child is exploiting the relationship with their carers, but really it is no more than comparing the experience which results (punishment or reward, a frown and a sharp word or a smile and encouraging words) against a prediction.

And what is true of this relatively conscious behaviour is also true of the child's nervous system as a whole. As with the process of detecting key features of the environment such as edges, changes in colour and movement, which speed up processing and learning, the brain operates by comparing experience to new events, predictions to what actually happens.

When you are about to get under the shower, you have a whole set of predictions about how it will feel based on past experience. You will usually concentrate on just one aspect of the barrage of sensory input that will result – is the water temperature right? This is the most important thing if you're not to get burnt or hit by a cold shock that will be very unpleasant. If you had to discriminate the temperature changes consciously, by processing all the other sensory input about the shower, it might take several minutes.

Taking a shower isn't usually a life-threatening exercise (aside from some classic horror movie scenes), but avoiding an approaching bus as we are crossing the road is critical. We have to be able to act fast to recognise that this is a bus and that it is coming towards us, without taking time to consider the situation.

By the end of the first 1,000 days of life, the child has usually developed some quite complex aspects of perception and behaviour. To a degree, they have understood what psychologists call the 'theory of mind'. This simply means that, while you may be feeling and thinking something – perhaps how boring the company of a particular person is right now – other people not only have thoughts and feelings of their own but they may be aware of yours as well. So it may not be in your best interest to show how bored you are, as it may just provoke anger which may make the situation worse.

As we get older, we can't function well as social beings without unconscious use of this theory of mind. The extent to which it is fundamental to a person's behaviour, and how strong their unconscious sense of this theory is, varies. In individuals with Asperger's syndrome for example it seems to be weaker and they may seem to find some social interactions difficult or they may behave inappropriately. This isn't necessarily a problem, especially once it has been recognised, because it is often counterbalanced by other skills and attributes.

Self-Control

Some aspects of self-control are conscious, and some happen whether we like it or not. What is becoming clear is that, like other aspects of brain function, self-control is set up in response to the world around us and starts in each of us before we are two years old.

The fact that it develops early in life suggests that a sense of self-control is important for the growing child. This is obviously important from a purely physical point of view, if toilet training is to be successful for example. The child has to learn that they must get to the toilet in good time.

Perhaps in fact, the development of a sense of time and of continuity underlies self-control more generally. If the child does not understand that a favourite food will still be there in a few minutes time, perhaps when other family members have had a chance to join the table, why not grab it now? And while having antiseptic cream and a plaster applied to a cut may make the cut hurt even more right now, there is no point in screaming and fighting because it will feel better in a few minutes.

Psychologists have been able to show that even young children can exercise self-control to a degree. For example, they can delay eating a treat for some time in order to get a bigger treat later. So self-control is already linked to a sense of time and to the consequences which an action now may have later. This is similar to the 'if-then' syntax (code) which is fundamental to computer programs. Parents or carers use this format without thinking: 'If you do that again, then I will take the toy away' or 'If you eat this vegetable up, then you can have your sweet'.

. Put together with the sense of the theory of mind, we can see how human social interactions develop: 'If I do that, then mummy will be cross. She'll be cross because she knows that I know I shouldn't do it'.

Will the child improve their behaviour as a result of understanding 'cause and effect', or decide to be deliberately naughty? Time and experience will tell

---

Behind this scenario lies a sense of cause and effect.

Will the child improve their behaviour as a result of understanding 'cause and effect', or decide to be deliberately naughty? Time and experience will tell.

This process of learning from our experience also operates for the motor, or movement controlling aspects of the brain. Drinking from a cup is a perilous business for a small child. But as adults, when we pick up a cup of hot coffee, we have (unconsciously) an idea of what it will weigh and where to hold it. As our fingers close around the handle, we predict that it will feel just like a handle; then the muscles of the arm contract to raise the cup in a smooth motion in three dimensions towards our lips. We will sip very cautiously at first and put the cup down if it's too hot or doesn't taste right.

Drinking coffee would be agonisingly slow if we had to consciously judge the weight of the cup, the need to keep it upright and the need to move it in three dimensions. The growing child's brain has to learn all this, from the important aspects of the sensory world to focus on, to the amount of force needed and the control necessary to carry out an action.

For adults, the developmental progress of a baby over the first two years can sometimes seem agonisingly slow. A new parent might long for the time when their child's bladder is under control, or the first steps are taken, or the first drink is taken from that cup. It can be frustrating waiting for these accomplishments to develop and hard to tell ourselves that most kids won't wear a nappy for life, will eventually walk and won't keep drinking from a baby bottle as an adult.

The good news is that usually this frustration is forgotten – when we ask older parents how long it took before their child, now grown up, could eat from a spoon unaided, for example, they usually can't remember.

But even so we can't resist the temptation of trying to accelerate the progress. We don't expect a young child to drink from a glass, but we assess how their sensory perception and motor control develop in order to decide what is appropriate – moving perhaps from a plastic trainer cup with a secure lid, to a small beaker and eventually to a glass itself. This is all part of the interaction process. As the child learns new skills, the kind of support they need changes too. What does not change is the need for positive encouragement.

Square Eyes

There's much interest, but also considerable concern, about the effects of the digital world on the development of young children. As with other aspects of their learning, in the first two years of life today's children learn very fast to use touch screens, a computer mouse and even a keyboard.

Devices and functions which are alien and hard to understand for older people are mastered effortlessly by young children. They seem to use them 'naturally'. This is to be expected: it's their world and they haven't known anything different. But as their brains learn quickly to use smartphones and laptops, we may wonder what the longer-term effects on their bodies and their brains will be.

Some effects are unsurprising. Children who spend hours playing computer games or just watching TV rather than engaging in physical activities are more likely to become overweight. And the light emitted by some tablets and laptops can stimulate the brain's system for distinguishing night from day and make it harder to get them to sleep at bedtime. But are there longer-term effects? We just don't know.

Some researchers think that the use of touch screens, which requires quite delicate, accurately controlled movements, will speed up and improve the development of hand–eye coordination. So will today's children grow up to be better at graphic art or tennis?

Others worry that a shift away from three-dimensional and conceptual skill development, such as the pastimes of their grandparents when they were children – gluing models together, needlework or domestic science – will delay or reduce acquisition of other aspects of fine movement control. So will today's children be unable to become brain surgeons?

But over one aspect of this brave new world all child development experts are agreed.

The potential exposure of even young children to graphic images, from violence to pornography, on the internet is a real danger. So is the risk of grooming by predators on social media. We clearly have to find effective ways of protecting children from these aspects of the digital world, and we also have to develop ways to educate them from an early age about such risks and about how to detect them and defend themselves.

Learning to Protect Yourself

We watch and marvel at how young children develop skills based on experience of the world, but there are many aspects of this which we can't see. The whole body is engaged in it – the growing cells, organs and systems. One which we increasingly realise to be very important is the immune system. This has to defend the body against foreign invaders, such as bacteria or viruses, throughout life. It does this by producing the body's equivalent of a missile defence system, antibodies which bind to the invaders and signal to special killer cells that they have found such invaders.

Like the visual system, the immune system has to refine its activities to be efficient. It can't just attach killer cells in the body without good reason. So it has to learn how to recognise something as foreign, to distinguish between 'self' and 'non-self'. To a certain extent, as with the visual system, this is an inborn property of the immune system but, as with the visual system it also depends on learning from experience.

For the fetus, in the relatively germ-free environment of the womb there isn't much opportunity to experience or learn about 'non-self', so really the learning exercise is largely around recognition of 'self'. The fetus in the womb is developing the thymus gland at the base of the neck which produces the immune cells. After birth the immune cells are produced by the bone marrow and the thymus has a smaller role. Life after birth is full of germs, and now the immune system will have to learn about a much wider range of targets.

So the baby is born with a degree of 'innate' immunity. The cells which are ready to detect foreign invaders ignore the other cells in the baby's blood, even though they are characterised by a particular blood group and would, if present in the bloodstream of a baby with a different blood group, produce an intense and very dangerous reaction.

From now on, the baby has to acquire the immunity on which its life may depend. When it meets invaders, for example the viruses which produce the common cold or COVID-19, its immune system gears up to tackle them by making antibodies to the virus and activating the killer cells. This usually takes several days, after which the infection begins to subside. Then the infant feels better, except that, just as in the adult, the viral infection is usually followed by a bacterial infection which makes pus in the nose and throat and could lead to a chest infection.

As doctors have learned during the pandemic, infection with COVID-19 can lead to a viral pneumonia which can be very dangerous. However, for reasons which have not yet been explained, the really dangerous consequences of COVID-19 infection are rare in young children.

Once exposed, the immune system has learned a strategy for dealing with a particular virus, and this is why when a nasty cold is circulating the infant won't catch it twice. When the virus invades again, the immune system is ready for it and will remember this virus pretty much for the rest of life. It is so effective that for some invaders, such as the measles virus, the immunity from future infection is complete.

We can induce this immunity by giving a weakened strain of the virus or bacteria to the child, by vaccination. This is now standard practice for the triple vaccine, MMR (mumps, measles and rubella). It is really important that all children receive this vaccine so that the population as a whole is immune to these dangerous and sometimes deadly organisms. This is the idea of 'herd immunity' which has been discussed repeatedly during the COVID-19 pandemic.

There were scare stories some years ago about the potentially harmful effects on the child's brain development from the MMR vaccination. They were unfounded but, sadly, some parents feel that they would rather not take the risk for their child. This isn't just being cautious – it's actually dangerous for them and their community. The unvaccinated child may catch measles, mumps or rubella and the diseases can spread very quickly throughout the population. The infections can be fatal in elderly people, affect male fertility and can produce deafness in a baby if a woman catches it while she is pregnant. We may not like to think of ourselves as part of a herd, but the reality is that no-one is safe until everyone is safe, so achieving and maintaining herd immunity can be argued to be everyone's duty.

The reason why these diseases don't make national news every day is because they are now rare. And they are rare because in most developed countries we have a high level of herd immunity because almost everyone is vaccinated. In some communities where the vaccination rate has dropped, we are now beginning to see these diseases becoming part of life, just as they were 100 years ago in the UK. In addition to this, our increased travel, destruction of wild environments and increased contact with wild animal species is leading to epidemics of diseases transmitted from animals to humans. They include AIDS, SARS, MERS, Zika and of course COVID-19 which at the time of writing has already infected more than 250 million people and caused the premature death of more than five million people globally.

There is another aspect of the environment about which the baby's immune system is also learning. Some components of that environment can produce a violent allergic reaction in some of us. We probably all know someone who is allergic to nuts, or eggs, or to certain pets. And conditions like asthma can be very distressing and even life-threatening in some people. Breathing problems like this can be triggered by house dust, which contains mites whose droppings the body recognises as foreign. Some of these allergies are increasingly common, and research shows that part of the problem is that many children are brought up in much cleaner environments than they were before – no dust, no animal hairs and certainly no animal droppings.

When we think of the conditions to which children were exposed even 100 years ago – in dusty and dirty urban environments for example or on farms in rural areas, the places where they played and even their schools – we can imagine that they were exposed to a barrage of potential pathogens. Of course, many childhood infectious diseases occurred as a result, and sadly childhood mortality was high. In 1920 nearly a third of the world's children died before they reached the age of five years.

But on the other hand, allergies and asthma were much less common. The immune systems of these children learned early in their lives to recognise these dirty aspects of the environment and to prepare defences against them.

Today, 'dirt' can come as a surprise to our children's bodies and produce an excessive reaction. No-one is suggesting living in squalor, but perhaps it doesn't make sense to be too clean? It is interesting that similar immune system reactions can happen to food and the current advice to parents and carers is to expose babies from about four to six months to some potential allergens such as peanuts or eggs. The baby, of course, isn't old enough to eat these things, and giving them whole nuts would pose a very dangerous risk of choking, but the amounts needed to help the immune system to learn are really very tiny.

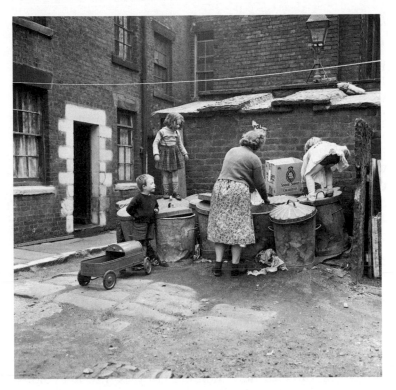

Figure 1.5 Children playing in dirty conditions in the 1960s
The immune systems of children learn from exposure to their environment and prepare defences. In current times, 'dirt' can come as a surprise to our children's bodies and produce an excessive reaction.
Mirrorpix/Getty Images.

One of the reasons why breastfeeding is recommended whenever possible is that breast milk contains some of the antibodies which the baby needs to protect itself. Getting this ready-made supply can also help to protect against infections at a time when the baby's immune system has not learned to recognise invaders. The other reason of course is that breast milk contains the complete set of nutrients that the baby needs.

Gut Instinct

Before we leave the immune system, there is another aspect of the foreign environment which we need to highlight. The environment in which we live isn't only outside us – it is inside our bodies too. From the mouth to the anus, our digestive systems are in fact part of the external world, basically a tube passing through us. The food we eat does not instantly become part of us – it remains in this tube while it is digested and only then are some of its constituents such as sugars, protein components and fats, absorbed into our bloodstream.

Our digestive system, the part of the external world which we carry around in us all the time, is populated by bacteria. There are in fact more bacteria in our guts than there are cells in the rest of our bodies, so we might say that we're really just walking homes for them. Fortunately, these bacteria are almost all useful to us. They help to digest our food, crowd our guts making it harder for other invaders to get a foothold, and can also influence our immune responses. Every day we pass billions of them out in our faeces, only for new members of this internal colony to breed and replace them.

Our 'microbiome', as this internal world of bacteria is called, is unique to each of us in some respects. We have literally inherited some members of it at birth, when we are inevitably exposed to our mother's body. We pick up some founder members of our gut microbiome at this time and they start to colonise the gut. Babies born by caesarean section will have a slightly different microbiome from those who are born vaginally for this reason, as will babies born to mothers who have recently taken a course of antibiotics. We'll return to the issue of delivering a baby and interventions like caesarean sections in Chapter 2.

Research on the microbiome is one of the most active and exciting areas in biology and medicine, and no doubt new discoveries about how 'friendly' bacteria affect our lives will soon be discovered. As we grow and develop, and learn about our world, the populations of bacteria within us are changing – learning too in a way – and these bacteria are going to influence how we respond to many aspects of our lives including the food we eat.

The End of the Beginning

As parents, as we look back on the time up to the child's second birthday, we often realise that many of our worries about the baby's development during that time were unfounded.

Probably the most common concern of parents or carers is about whether the infant is growing well. Much time and effort are spent on weighing infants and plotting their growth on a chart to see how well it conforms to that expected, on the basis of data for the population as a whole. It is true that the babies who struggle with their health and wellbeing during infancy are the babies who aren't growing well. Poor growth is a marker of problems, but growth charts also cause a good deal of unnecessary anxiety.

We also worry about babies who are growing rather too fast for the population graph, because they're often becoming too fat. We know that the risk of obesity in childhood, and then in teenagers and adults, can start in the first 1,000 days of life, and this is something we'll return to later in the book.

Some things come naturally to the baby, and in many ways, they are far more in control of their lives than we might think

---

Some things come naturally to the baby, and in many ways, they are far more in control of their lives than we might think.

One of the great advantages of breastfeeding is that it is impossible to overfeed the baby. The baby will detach from the nipple when they've had enough, and breast milk contains the perfect combination of nutrients. Some infant formulas can provide too much nutrition, which may not always be balanced, and it is too easy to overfeed an infant by using a bottle.

But society does not always make it easy for the nature of the baby to exert itself. Support for breastfeeding, for example by providing clean safe rooms for women who wish to feed their babies when they are outside the home, are not available in many places, whether public or private. As well, there are many experiences of a healthcare system which is under-resourced to provide the breastfeeding support that is needed. Many women talk of the pressure put on them to breastfeed, while sometimes this isn't possible for many reasons, leading to feelings of guilt or failure as mothers.

But in the next phase of the infant's feeding even more potential problems are encountered. Weaning is a time for more decisions and influence by parents with the introduction of solid foods. It's a time when the baby needs more robust sources of food, and when they can start to experience new flavours and textures. It is also a time when an unhealthy diet can increase the risk of the child becoming overweight or obese. Parents need support, because some weaning foods can be unbalanced in nutritional terms and provide excessive calories.

JM Barrie once said: 'You always know after you are two. Two is the beginning of the end'. *He might have been reading this book*

So the moment-to-moment response of body and behaviour to the environment of a child, and the learning that takes place, will influence that child's development.

We may not be able to recall anything about our first two years, but our bodies and brains have in-built memories which will shape our future lives. This was appreciated by the author JM Barrie, who created the character Peter Pan, the boy who could fly and who inspired many other children's entertainments such as pantomimes. But Peter Pan never grew up in the stories. There is a clinical condition, called Peter Pan syndrome, which describes adults who want to remain infantile.

Barrie once said: 'You always know after you are two. Two is the beginning of the end'. He might have been reading this book – and discovered how important our first two years are.

But JM Barrie's idea is somewhat fatalistic – as if the game was over at the age of two. We disagree, and believe that an optimistic view is nearer the truth. We would say that age two in many ways marks the *end of the beginning* of making a person, the phase when what our bodies and our brains have 'learned' sets the course for our best chances in life. So, as we are telling the story of our development backwards, we need to go back further in time if we are to understand that beginning. We need to think about our lives in the womb. And that immediately faces us with one of the greatest challenges we meet in the whole of our lives – being born.

2 A NARROW ESCAPE

On the Rocks

Images scraped into the rocks many hundreds of years ago by First Nation people living near what is now the town of Moab, in the US state of Utah, show a multitude of animals and birds. But also give rare glimpses into the everyday lives of the people who made these images, including the image in Figure 2.1.

It depicts a person spread-eagled on the rock, with what can only be a baby emerging between their legs. The baby is very large compared to the mother, and is perhaps exaggerated, but it suggests a very difficult birth, possibly with fatal consequences for both the mother and the baby. Is that why this everyday event was recorded?

Other cultures have recorded similar potentially tragic events. A sculpture on the tomb of a Greek mother from about 340 BCE shows her bidding farewell to her husband as she dies in childbirth. Childbirth, with a happy outcome or not, was so common that it was seldom recorded unless the woman or her family were wealthy.

If we go forward to a time only about 120 years ago when modern obstetric care in childbirth had not been developed, we discover that maternal mortality even in rich countries was about 50 per 1,000 births. And the number of babies who died at birth or in the first week of life was similar.

In the absence of reliable contraception, and with such high infant mortality, many women for thousands of years

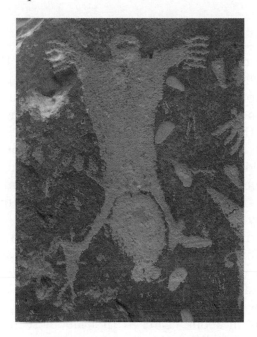

Figure 2.1 Giving birth is as old as the hills
An ancient image carved into a rock panel
on public land administered by the Bureau
of Land Management near Moab, Utah,
USA. It appears to represent a woman
giving birth.
Photograph by Mark Hanson.

had a series of pregnancies at one- to two-year intervals
throughout their reproductive lives – and their lives might
be quite short as a result. Deaths were common even in
women who seemed fit and healthy throughout pregnancy, so there did not seem to be much which could be
done to prevent these commonplace tragedies.

Ordinary motherhood required extraordinary courage.
But pregnancy and childbirth are still very risky even in
countries with good medical care. Why is that? We can see
some of the challenges if we follow one woman's case history, provided in the box.

No Ordinary Birth

Rachel's first pregnancy was at the age of 29. Her baby grew well and all seemed to be going according to plan.

By about 34 weeks of pregnancy the fetus should have done a somersault in the womb and engaged its head in the pelvis ready to be born head first. Rachel's baby was certainly an active fetus, and she thought that she could feel it kicking quite forcefully in her pelvis. The bulge at the top of her womb did not seem to have become smaller either. So she was fairly convinced that her baby had not performed its somersault and was still moving around with the head uppermost. She discussed this with the midwife at her 34-week antenatal assessment but, after feeling her abdomen, the midwife dismissed this concern.

One week later, she went into labour on a Saturday night at about 11pm. At first labour seemed to be progressing well but then, at about 6.30am on Sunday morning it was clear that the process had stopped. The external monitor placed on her abdomen wasn't showing strong contractions of her uterus and the fetal heart rate recording seemed unsteady. The midwife and colleagues on duty decided that a better recording of the heart rate was essential to assess whether the baby was OK.

Rachel's cervix, the passage between the womb and the outside world, was dilated several centimetres, and the skin of what appeared to be the baby's head could be clearly seen. This would allow a scalp electrode to be attached directly to the baby, to give a more reliable recording of its heart rate. When this was connected to the monitor it still did not give a stable signal, and it seemed to show that the baby's heart rate was about 80 beats per minute. This is about half the value expected for a healthy fetus around the time of birth.

Clearly something was wrong. There was no reason to think that the monitor was faulty and the connection of the scalp electrode seemed OK. If the baby's heart rate really was as low as this then it could be a sign of fetal distress. Further action was needed. The obstetrician on duty was called in to give an opinion. He wasn't happy about Rachel's baby having a heart rate half of what it should be. It needed to be delivered fast.

Quickly, he was able to get a grip through the cervix of what had been supposed to be the baby's head, which turned out to be a *foot*. This was a so-called 'breech' delivery. This explained why the heart monitor wasn't working properly as it is designed to pick up the heartbeat from the scalp, not the sole of the foot. A bit of manipulation allowed him to deliver the baby feet-first. The baby, a girl, let out a strong cry. Clearly she was fine.

Breech deliveries occur in around 4% of pregnancies and these days they should be safe. But in the past they would have been dangerous, especially if the baby's bottom had to be delivered first or a leg became trapped. If the legs are delivered first, as with Rachel's baby, it's called a 'footling' breech.

Perhaps it's fair to say that anything could happen at birth. There are 'no ordinary births' but, thanks to speedy action by health professionals, family and other birthing support, most births have a happy outcome.

There are 135 million babies born every year in the world. And around the world about 840 women die every day from complications related to pregnancy – that's more than one death every two minutes. Their babies, even if they survive, are already motherless. And for every woman who dies, about 20–30 more suffer from physical trauma or other problems which can have lifelong consequences.

Even in the twenty-first century every birth is an expedition into the unknown. Take for example the USA, the country which spends more on healthcare than any other. Maternal mortality in the USA was just over 17 deaths per 100,000 live births in 2018, and has actually increased since the year 2000. Worse still, the figure among Black women was more than double this, at 37 deaths per 100,000 live births. The pattern seems similar, or worse, in the UK, with mortality in Black women four times higher, and that of Asian women twice that of White women.

In both the USA and UK death associated with childbirth is more common in Black women

---

In many low-income countries, where resources are poor and medical support is very limited, the monitoring and intervention that we described in Rachel's case don't exist. Even after the successful delivery of a healthy baby, blood loss or infection claim the lives of many women. The deaths often happen because the woman already had a medical condition, such as high blood pressure, which had not been recognised. Poor health is likely to be the cause of the greater mortality in Black women in the USA, and may also be linked to poorer overall healthcare.

These deaths are almost all preventable but clearly depend on where you are and what barriers exist to healthcare. But globally, thanks to enormous efforts on the part of healthcare professionals, government and international organisations and educationalists, the number of these maternal deaths fell by nearly 40% in the first 17 years of this millennium. Progress now may be much slower due to the impact of the COVID-19 pandemic in directing resources away from maternity care and lockdown measures making it more difficult for women to access this care.

In the case of obstructed labour, when the fetus is effectively stuck and can't be born without medical intervention, lack of such help can lead to fetal death. The mother may have tearing of her genito-urinary tract or rectum leaving her incontinent, and this can sometimes lead to her being socially excluded. Teams of volunteer doctors have worked tirelessly in some countries such as Ethiopia to find these women and to repair the damage to their bodies so that they can return to a more normal life.

The risk of such birthing problems is greatly increased in cultures where the custom of female genital mutilation still exists, which can sometimes involve stitching of the labia, the lips that protect the opening to the vagina. This is one form of sexual violence against women. It is highly appropriate that the 2018 Nobel Peace Prize was awarded to Dr Dennis Mukwege from the Democratic Republic of Congo, a gynaecologist who has worked tirelessly for years to repair the damage to women who have suffered from this and other forms of sexual violence.

Nor is the infant safe. In England and Wales nearly four babies out of every 1,000 born die in the perinatal (around birth) period, and many more are harmed as a result of a prolonged or difficult labour during which their brains did not receive enough oxygen.

Not all births happen in hospital. Every year in the UK 13,500 women choose to give birth at home, some with midwife support, support from family or non-medically qualified birth companions like a Doula, and some without any support at all. Other European countries vary in the fraction of women who have home births.

Usually, birth proceeds smoothly and does not require medical attention or intervention. But a birth at home may turn out to need more medical assistance than was anticipated and all high-income countries have arrangements in place for such intervention if needed. This might involve an urgent transfer to hospital for an epidural anaesthetic for the mother, help delivering the baby using instruments, or a caesarean section.

Similarly, a birth in hospital which a couple had hoped would take place in a birthing pool may in the end take place in an operating theatre. A woman who had thought that the only thing she would need to blunt the pain would be to breathe gas and air, a mixture containing the analgesic nitrous oxide, may be faced with an epidural anaesthetic injected around the spinal cord in the lower back to block pain altogether. Or a woman who had wanted the maximum amount of medication to reduce pain may find that birth progresses so fast that there is no time for that.

Who's in Control?

At the end of the day (or night) the process of birth is the province of the mother. The woman's partner may be present, to support her, but can't take on the job themself. They are not in control.

Many cultures across the world have had, even in recent times, a tradition where the male partner attempts to go through the process of labour. This practice, called *couvade*, has been documented from ancient times. The details vary, but usually it involves the woman leaving the 'childbed' and the male partner taking her place, to writhe and moan, acting out the process of labour and delivery. When the baby is actually born to the mother, it may be given to him to comfort and he may even pretend to breastfeed it. In some cultures, where there are dietary restrictions for the mother after delivery, the father will go through these too.

Needless to say, then it's the male partner who receives congratulations and presents. We won't dwell on this, but you can imagine that opinions are divided even among anthropologists and social historians about *couvade*. Is it an example of a patriarchal desire to retain control over the woman's body and gain ownership of the child? Or is it a necessary device to ensure that men empathise with their partners and engage in the responsibilities of fatherhood from Day One? There continues to be a fascination with this, some websites documenting use of transcutaneous electrical nerve stimulation (TENS) technology to simulate childbirth for men.

There are many lessons which could be learned from Rachel's case history we described earlier, starting with 'always listen to the mother'. Adhering to a strict protocol during the birth procedure, with rules about when to change plans, is also clearly very important.

Monitoring contractions and the baby's heart rate during birth helps medical staff to decide if and when to intervene. They may need to call for more powerful anaesthesia, a caesarean section or delivery of the baby with instruments, ranging from a suction device to forceps placed around the baby's head. These interventions usually have to be made by a doctor – an obstetrician, rather than a midwife.

There has always been an element of taboo, if not embarrassment, about these interventions, as if somehow using them meant that the birth was not 'natural'. Even in the sixteenth century, when doctors – who of course were usually men, the so-called 'man-midwives' – developed such interventions, there was an element of secrecy involved. The forceps they used, which look like large tongs for a domestic fire, had handles covered in leather so that they did not make a noise, and were usually hidden under a cloth.

Some couples go to great lengths to stage-manage the birth of their baby, wanting this to be a wonderful experience for all concerned. They plan what to eat, the background music that they'll play, the lighting and any special pillows or gadgets that they'll take along. They naturally want to 'take control' of this important event.

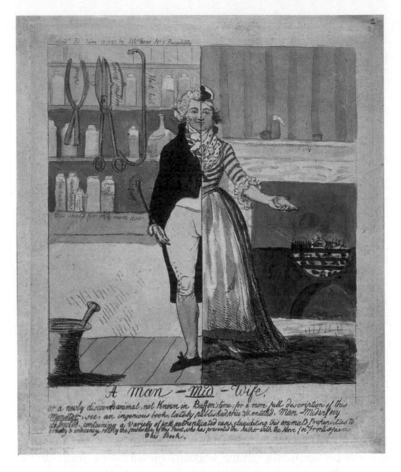

Figure 2.2 Man-midwife This etching from the late eighteenth century was a protest against male birth assistants and the danger they posed to female modesty and virtue.
A 'man-midwife' (male obstetrician) is represented by a figure divided in half, one half representing a man and the other half a woman.
Coloured etching by I. Cruikshank, 1793. Wellcome Collection.

Are they focussed on birth as a beginning of a new chapter of life, or as the endpoint or finale to the present one? After all, there is a big build-up to birth so it may well feel like a finale.

There is so much emphasis on health and lifestyle in pregnancy; so many websites giving information; so many chatrooms for sharing experiences; and so much advice from friends, family, colleagues etc. This can be quite overwhelming and stressful for prospective parents, especially because the information available online can be contradictory.

We'll come back to questions of parental responsibility later in the book. Any approach a couple take to planning or managing the birth of their baby can leave a potential nagging feeling that this was not the right decision. But all couples should realise that, however carefully laid their plans for the birth, they may well have to be abandoned. The birth may have been different from their plans, but it is no less significant.

Exit Strategy

During the last third of pregnancy, the fetus appears to be fine-tuning its development and getting ready to be born. It's finalising the number of heart muscle cells it will have for the rest of its life, completing the development of the branching tree of tubes in its lungs ready to breathe air, laying down muscle and bone in its limbs, putting fat cells in place and filling some of them with fat to give it some thermal insulation and an energy store for its early life outside the womb.

We'll discuss these developments in the next chapter. But even though it continues to increase in size, the rate of growth of the baby is slowing in these final stages of pregnancy. The placenta, which formed at the end of the first part of pregnancy, and which has served it in terms of food and oxygen supply and removal of waste products, is now not large enough to support a great deal more growth. The end of this part of its first 1,000 days must be near.

But who makes the next move; who decides when birth happens?

Research over recent years has shown that the fetus is much more in control of its growth and development than we used to think. If it grew too large to pass physically through the birth canal, then all the effort and resource which both it and its mother have put into the process over the last nine months would be wasted. We've already seen the risk that this would pose to it and its mother's life. So there has to be some compromise now, as there will be in so many of the relations between the baby and its mother later.

It is part of the fetal brain, the pituitary gland, which sends out the hormonal signal through its blood stream to initiate the birth process – the uterine contractions of labour. For humans, the timing of this is more variable than it is in many animals. In the sheep for example, the length of pregnancy is usually about 147 days and varies by only a few days, and in rats it is 21 days and it often happens at night. In humans the situation is very different, with labour starting anywhere between 37 and 42 weeks of pregnancy considered as normal, and birth happening at any time of the day or night.

If a baby is born before 37 weeks of gestation, it is considered to be born preterm. There may be concerns about whether organs such as its lungs have matured sufficiently – it may need special care, perhaps in a neonatal intensive care unit. Conversely, after 42 weeks, the concern might be that the placenta is becoming too old to meet the demands of the fetus. The variability in the timing of the start of labour may be the result of the complex interactions which have to take place between the fetus, the placenta and the mother in preparation for birth.

Even though there are some spontaneous contractions of the muscles of the mother's uterus in the last weeks of pregnancy, these will have been uncoordinated and not very forceful. For the baby to be expelled from the uterus, the muscular contractions have to start at the top of the uterus and pass in forceful waves downwards. At the same time, the tissues of the cervix have to become softer and more stretchable, switching from a sphincter that keeps the baby, placenta and amniotic sac all within the womb, to an expandable channel through which the baby and then the placenta can pass.

The process of birth represents a truly joint 'decision' by the fetus and the mother

So the initiation of the process of birth represents a truly joint 'decision' by the fetus and the mother. Once the decision has been made, a cascade of hormonal changes takes place in the placenta which drives all the preparatory steps necessary for labour and delivery of the baby.

The adrenal glands of the fetus, located just above its kidneys, are almost as big as the kidneys themselves at this time in life. They have a special zone, which will disappear after birth. This fetal zone makes hormones important for fetal development and birth. One such adrenal hormone is cortisol, usually thought of as a stress hormone, which is essential for the final maturation stages of fetal organs such as the lungs. It is also important for making the hormone progesterone by the placenta, which prevents the mother ovulating and maintains her pregnancy. Another adrenal hormone, called dehydroepiandrosterone, is also secreted into the bloodstream, and is then altered as it passes through the fetal liver and then converted in the placenta to oestrogen. As its levels rise towards birth it plays its part in how other pregnancy hormones work, developing the organs of the fetus and placenta and developing the mother's breast tissue ready to produce milk.

Changes in these hormones are kick-started by a hormone signal from the fetal pituitary gland at the base of its brain. The pituitary is the master controller of hormones in the body. But starting the physical process of birth requires the mother's hormonal systems to be ready to play their part, and the metabolic machinery of the placenta has to be ready too.

Best Laid Plans

This seems like a good system. For the vast majority of the 135 million births that occur every year around the world, it is, and the process leads to a happy outcome. All the birth planning works out and the event is just as the parents and family had hoped. But, as in Rachel's case, medical attention or intervention may be needed, and quickly.

Now that we've thought about the processes involved in being born, we can perhaps explain why this common occurrence, an essential part of all of our lives, is so dangerous in our species.

There are several purely mechanical explanations for this danger: there is nothing subtle about them. One is the big head of the fetus which we mentioned earlier. The human brain is very large, contained in our large skull, and most of the development of the brain has taken place before birth. The passage of the baby's head through the birth canal means that it has to squeeze through the tunnel formed by the bones of the mother's pelvis. These are joined at the front by cartilage, which allows the bony tunnel to stretch, but not by much.

In addition, the tunnel is not uniform in its shape, so the baby's head has to start passing through it facing to right or left. Then, before it can exit, the head must turn to face either directly forwards or backwards. This is quite a complex manoeuvre. Finally, exit itself depends on the forceful contractions of the uterus and the softening of the cervix to allow the baby to pass through.

There is nothing the baby can do to help – fetal movements stop before labour. So it cannot turn its head itself, or help its exit by struggling or kicking – just as well because it could cause damage

---

There is nothing the baby can do to help – and in fact fetal movements stop before labour. So it cannot turn its head itself, or help its exit by struggling or kicking, which is perhaps just as well because it would be more likely to hinder the process or cause damage.

Being born head first means that the largest part of the baby has to get through the birth canal first. It's like the thick end of a wedge, but it makes sense. It gives the baby the best chance of being able to get some air as quickly as possible. Also, the baby is less likely to get stuck; trying to push a leg, an arm or a shoulder through is much more likely to involve the baby's awkward shape getting jammed.

Another of the mechanical dangers of the birth process is that the umbilical cord can become trapped, cutting off the baby's supply of oxygen. It may be squashed against the side of the birth canal, or a loop may be pushed down through the canal, or the baby may even have the cord wrapped round its neck like a scarf.

The heart and brain of the fetus are very resilient to the potentially damaging effects of lack of oxygen, at least compared to later in life. The baby can sometimes be manoeuvred, and the mother can change her birthing position, to relieve some pressure on the umbilical cord. But at this time the midwives and doctors need to move quickly to avoid the supply being cut off for too long with the consequent risk of brain damage.

Even during normal delivery, the forceful contractions of the uterus can compress the cord, reducing the oxygen supply to the fetus for some minutes. The fetus responds to this by slowing down its heart rate, as this is a simple way to use less oxygen. This is quite normal, and once the contraction of the uterus subsides, the fetal heart rate should increase again promptly. If it does not, this may be a sign that the fetus is struggling to get enough oxygen for most of the time, not just during uterine contractions.

This was the concern in the case of Rachel's baby we discussed earlier. Maybe the cord was partially trapped, or perhaps the placenta had started to detach from the inner wall of the uterus too soon. This is why the midwife or obstetrician observed very carefully the pattern of contractions and the fetal heart rate responses as they were displayed in real time on a chart recorder, and were prepared to take swift action when the baby's heart was possibly signalling danger. But, as we saw, this all depends on the correct placement and use of the monitoring equipment. Accidents can happen and even mistakes can sometimes be made.

When there seems to be a problem developing during the process of labour and delivery of the fetus, midwives and doctors have to decide whether to let the mother and fetus battle on, or whether to press the 'Emergency Exit button' and opt for a rapid caesarean section, for example.

So decisions which can have important consequences have to be made rapidly. Press the Exit button too soon, when it may not have been necessary, and they will deprive the mother of the experience of a natural birth and leave her with more pain and a post-operative recovery which may make breastfeeding more difficult – let alone generate additional cost to the healthcare provider or health service. But waiting too long before acting may result in a brain-damaged baby who may have reduced quality of life and possibly need lifelong care.

The decision isn't an easy one and usually depends on a good deal of experience, shared between the team. It isn't surprising that the uterine contraction and fetal heart rate recordings made during birth often appear in cases of litigation when the question of whether the right decision was made is disputed.

The Compromise

When we think about all this, we can see why we are the only species on the planet which requires a birth assistant, someone to help a mother to deliver her baby. There are of course instances of a woman delivering her baby in isolation, on her own, but they are unusual and risky. We need help, and that need can become urgent quite rapidly.

In developed countries, or high resource settings, this usually means a medical assistant. It may be a primary healthcare physician or general practitioner (GP), a midwife or an obstetrician and team. Whoever it is, they have to be aware of a clearly defined protocol for what to do if it looks as if the delivery is not going well. In some places where giving birth at home is usual, there needs to be a plan for how to get the mother to hospital, or medical help brought to her, rapidly, if the need arises.

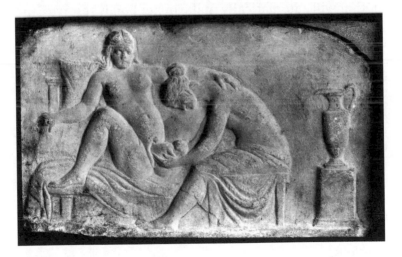

Figure 2.3 Assistance at birth in ancient Rome There are some purely mechanical reasons why we are the only species needing a birth assistant.
The ancient Roman relief carving shows a midwife attending a woman giving birth.
Wellcome Collection. Attribution 4.0 International (CC BY 4.0).

For humans it's crucial to deliver the head of the baby at birth. But the mechanical explanations we have described don't address the more fundamental 'why' question. Why in our fetal life do we grow heads which are almost too large to be born?

The answer lies way back in our evolutionary past as a species. It relates to a potential conflict between two aspects of our evolution. The first, clearly, is the evolution of a large brain, which marks our hominid ancestors out from other species. We believe, although of course we can never know for sure, that this accompanied our evolving skills in using our hands, inventing things and learning and communicating ideas and skills to our friends, family and children. Through this cultural evolution human society, arts, science and religious beliefs all developed. Perhaps the fundamentals of brain development evolved to take place before birth because, due to the sacrifices the mother will automatically make in her bodily reserves, nutrition is more secure in the womb than in the period after birth.

The second aspect of our evolution concerns the mother's body itself. A key phase in our evolution occurred when we started to walk upright on two legs. This may have given us an advantage as a species in being able to move from a forest to a savanna environment, because being upright enabled us to see game, predators or competing human groups some way off. Some other mammals which live in grassland environments, such a meerkats or mongoose, adopt a similar position by standing on their hind legs or sitting up on their haunches, but they can't hold the position for a long time and still have to run on four legs.

But walking and running upright as opposed to on all fours creates new mechanical challenges. The pelvis needs to rotate to allow our legs to be comfortably in line with the body. We can see this if we look at how awkward it is for a dog or a cat to stand on their hind legs for any length of time. In addition, standing upright means that the contents of the abdomen – the intestines, liver, uterus, bladder etc. – have to be supported by the pelvis rather than the front wall of the belly itself. This will be even more important if we start running, when these organs will bounce up and down. Preventing them descending necessitates narrowing of the pelvis.

The combined effect of evolving a large brain and a narrower pelvis is that the fetal head only just passes through the birth canal formed by the inner dimensions of the pelvis. Our nearest evolutionary cousins, the chimpanzees, move around mostly on four legs and so their pelvis is oriented for this.

The fetal chimp also has a smaller head relative to its body than we do. So birth is much easier for chimps.

It appears that during our evolution a conflict occurred between the need for a narrower, re-oriented pelvis which enabled us to walk upright and the advantage of growing a larger brain before birth. Evolution seems to have compromised, so that most babies can be born safely, and they and their mothers survive, even if some external help is often needed. Presumably if the maternal or infant mortality was unacceptably high, in terms of survival of the population, then there would have been an evolutionary advantage in developing slightly smaller brains and heads.

Give unto Caesar

Faced with the life-threatening situation of a woman in obstructed labour, a caesarean section may be the only course of action. The name comes from the myth that Julius Caesar was born by this method, although there is no historical record to confirm this, and in fact the name may really come from the Latin word *caedere* meaning 'to cut'. Caesarean section was practised long before anaesthesia

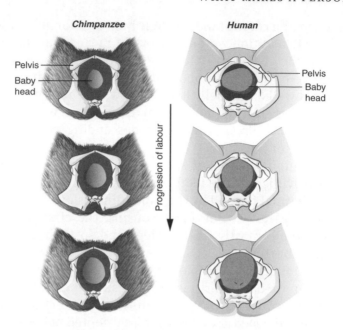

Figure 2.4 A tight squeeze For humans, the evolution to walking upright with a narrowing of the pelvis was at odds with our evolution of a bigger brain.

and antibiotics were developed. It was done to save the baby, and the mother would almost inevitably have died. Without the intervention both mother and baby would be expected to perish.

The procedure would never have been common, and was perhaps reserved for highly valued offspring such as those of monarchy. Perhaps this is why it was recorded. In Greek myth the God of Medicine, Asclepius, to whom many people prayed and left sacrifices in the hope of a safe birth or a cure from disease, was said to have been pulled from his mother's body by his father Apollo, the God of Music.

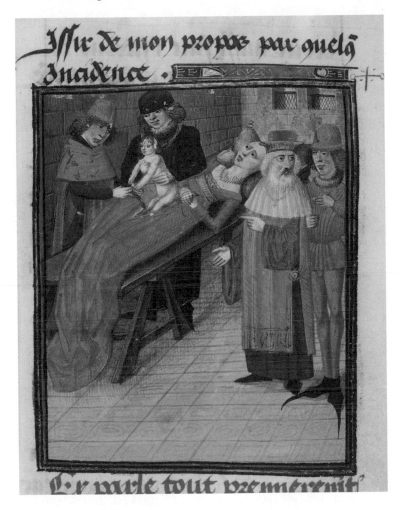

Figure 2.5 Birth by caesarian section This miniature from the illuminated manuscript *Bellum Gallicum* (*Les commentaires de Cesar*) 1473–1476 depicts the fabled delivery of baby Julius Caesar by a caesarean section. Now an increasingly common procedure, then it would almost certainly have been fatal for the woman.
The British Library, Royal 16 G VIII f. 32.

The idea of caesarean section has historically often had unnatural implications, perhaps because it involved effectively murder of the mother. In Shakespeare's play, Macbeth encounters three witches, stirring a ghastly concoction as it brews on a fire. He believes that they will be able to prophesy his destiny. One of their ghostly forms tells him that he will not be vanquished by any man 'of woman born'. So Macbeth feels safe enough – after all, how might he meet a foe who was not born to a woman?

It is not until later, in Act V of the play, that Macbeth meets MacDuff in battle, whom he discovers was 'from his mother's womb untimely ripped' – in other words delivered not vaginally but by caesarean section. Macbeth's fate is sealed.

With the advent of modern medical care – anaesthetics, antibiotics and aseptic surgical techniques – caesarean section became a very safe procedure. All the dangers of the fetal head having to squeeze through the pelvic birth canal and so obstruct labour, and the risk of the fetal brain being deprived of oxygen, are avoided.

If a doctor wanted to conduct a trial in which women were allowed to deliver babies vaginally, it is probable that no medical ethics committee would allow the trial to go ahead – it's just too dangerous!

An eminent obstetrician once remarked that if caesarean section were the standard normal mode of delivery but a doctor wanted to conduct a trial in which women were allowed to deliver babies vaginally, it is probable that no medical ethics committee would allow the trial to go ahead – it's just too dangerous!

Caesarean section is now the preferred mode of delivery for many couples in some parts of the world. For example, in some cities in Brazil and in parts of China more than

80% of babies are delivered by caesarean section. The rate is rising in many other countries too. There are many reasons for this trend beyond just safety considerations. It can be more convenient to decide in advance the timing of delivery for practical or cultural reasons and the pain and physical process of vaginal delivery are avoided. Sometimes there are even 'caesarean parties' organised so that several mothers can deliver their babies at the same time. The procedure can be popular with some obstetricians too, as they may charge for the procedure and can arrange their operating schedules in advance.

The cost of caesarean birth to healthcare systems is substantial, and it has limiting effects on the woman in the post-natal recovery period. In addition, the baby is of course born just a little before the cascade of hormonal and other signals which are involved in the normal process of labour, and so is not exposed to these processes. As we mentioned in Chapter 1, vaginal delivery also exposes the baby to the mother's microbiome and helps to populate its own gut with healthy bacteria. Data are just emerging about the effects of the microbiome on long-term health, so this may be very important if it isn't experienced with a caesarean birth.

Constrained Circumstances

Whatever the mode of delivery, once the baby is born one of the first things to happen is that it is weighed. At least that is what happens in high-income countries. Babies are typically a little larger in a woman's second and subsequent pregnancies than her first. Also, the size of babies at birth varies between ethnic groups. For example, in the UK, babies born to women of Indian, Pakistani and Bangladeshi ethnic background tend to be about 350 grams lighter than those of White ethnic background. There are many factors involved, but a smaller maternal stature is one.

But recent data which brings together the outcomes of more than a million pregnancies in England between 2015 and 2017 reveals much more worrying influences. Research showed that about 24% of the risk of stillbirths, 19% of the risk of preterm birth and 31% of the risk of having a baby with a low birthweight could be accounted for by socio-economic inequality for this population. When the researchers factored in the influences of ethnic group, smoking and obesity, the effects were much less, showing that the effects of low socio-economic level on birth outcomes could be largely driven by these factors. We'll return in Chapter 5 to the implications of such inequalities, but it is shocking to see such effects on the early lives of the next generation in a developed country which has a proud history of public health.

In the context of the Nature versus Nurture debate we discussed in Chapter 1, the impact of socio-economic factors on fetal growth emphasise that this cannot simply be a genetic (Nature) process. In addition, if it were, we would expect the father's genes inherited by the fetus to play as much of a role in influencing its growth as the mother's genes. This won't do, because it's the mother who has to grow the baby and give birth to it. So the elements of her genetic makeup which the fetus has inherited are more important in influencing her baby's size up until the time of birth. After that, the father's genes begin to play a role too, so that by the time their offspring is fully grown their height will usually be somewhere between the father's and the mother's height.

'Maternal constraint' limits the growth of the fetus to match the mother's stature, reflecting her body proportions

---

The process by which the mother limits the growth of her fetus before birth is called 'maternal constraint'. It limits the growth of the fetus to match her stature, reflect-ing her body proportions. In addition to suppressing the growth-promoting influences of the genetic information inherited from the father until after birth, there are also a range of other factors which influence the degree to which this maternal constraint acts.

Constraint is greater in first pregnancies, perhaps be-cause the uterus has not been stretched before, and per-haps because the blood supply to the placenta may not increase as much during a first pregnancy as during subse-quent ones. Constraint is greater in twins or triplets: they are crammed into a womb that can only expand a certain amount to accommodate them. Even though their com-bined weight at birth is greater than a single fetus, each of them is smaller than the average singleton.

Constraint is also greater if the mother is very young, for example still a teenager. This is perhaps because she is still growing her own body and so the question arises of how much of her available resources can be devoted to her growth, and how much to her growing fetus.

Evolutionary biologists argue that when there is a con-flict of interest like this, the mother must win: after all, she has survived to achieve reproductive success, and could conceive again. In contrast, her fetus is an untried and un-tested member of the species – it may not turn out to be a reproductively successful member of the species and so its role is more uncertain from an evolutionary point of view.

This is a very harsh, and simplistic, way of looking at development with which many of us would not agree. But whatever the truth of this, it is certain that the health and survival of both women and their babies is often poor in countries where girls may marry in their early teens and conceive their first child soon after. They may have little choice in the matter as contraception isn't always readily available or acceptable. The situation is sometimes made worse if they cease to attend school. The COVID pandemic has made this problem worse as it has prevented millions of women worldwide from having access to contraception, and also prevented school attendance in some settings.

These considerations have led bodies such as the WHO to recommend that girls should not become pregnant in their early teens. There are other considerations too. If pregnant women are expected to continue hard physical work such as agriculture or carrying water in large containers over long distances, we can imagine that the conflict between the energy needed for the mother to undertake this work and that required to grow her fetus can be stark. This is particularly true in late pregnancy, when the fetal demands are greatest and the mother's cardiovascular system is working hard to deliver supply. The situation may be made even worse if the mother's diet is poor, and in some societies women only eat after the men and other family members. Sometimes they are also expected to fast on one or more days each week.

Other types of maternal constraint are related to things that interfere with the woman's ability to pass nutrition to her fetus. The malaria parasite depends on a supply of iron, like most living organisms, so part of the body's defence against it is to reduce the absorption of iron from food by the gut. The result can be iron deficiency anaemia, in which the red blood cells contain smaller amounts of haemoglobin, the oxygen-carrying molecule which contains iron. This can reduce the transport of oxygen to the fetus, compromising its growth and development.

A somewhat similar problem occurs with women who smoke during pregnancy. Smoking alters the oxygen-carrying capacity of the blood and has been clearly shown to reduce fetal growth.

Looking at the factors which can effectively alter the level of maternal constraint of fetal growth, you might realise that many are associated with lower socio-economic status. These factors are likely to have played a part in influencing patterns of fetal growth during hard times for families at many periods of history.

Clear evidence that these processes are still operating comes from the effects of the global financial crisis of 2008. This was associated with an increase in the number of babies born with low birthweight in many countries. This is very unfortunate because it will increase their risk of chronic diseases later in life, with additional cost implications for them, their families and society. We'll discuss this more in Chapter 5.

Socio-economic crises and government policies of austerity, which often hit the poorest sections of the population hardest, thus perpetuate the cycle of poverty across generations and reduce chances of upward social mobility. The impact of the COVID-19 pandemic on the health of mothers and their children has been severe, and has been much greater than its effects on men. Since the onset of the pandemic, coverage of lifesaving health interventions for women, children and adolescents in 36 low- to middle-income countries has dropped by up to 25%. Four million pregnant women have lost access to childbirth care, there has been a 28% increase in the odds of a stillbirth and a 37% increase in the odds of maternal death.

But is this discussion getting out of hand? True, fetal growth will be challenged in women who smoke or who are unlucky enough to have some clinical condition such as pre-eclampsia or an infection such as malaria. But millions upon millions of pregnancies have taken place with very good results for hundreds of thousands of years. Shouldn't we focus our attention on these perfectly normal pregnancies, with their happy outcomes?

The answer of course is 'Yes', but that's just the point. From the practical point of view we've just explained, the processes of maternal constraint take place in every pregnancy, even all those that are completely normal and don't qualify as 'low birthweight'. We need to think about the possible consequences of this normal, but nonetheless under-recognised, process.

The processes of maternal constraint, where the mother limits the growth of her baby, take place in every pregnancy

---

The Bigger the Better?

To test the idea that maternal constraint does act on fetal growth even in a wide spectrum of normal babies, we can look at large datasets for healthy populations. With such data for over about 1.2 million births in the Netherlands between 2000 and 2008, we find as expected that birthweights varied, although most of the babies had weights around the average for this population. We might guess from all we've said earlier that the chances of survival were worse in the very smallest babies, and also the very largest babies. In a country such as the Netherlands with good healthcare, the number of the babies that this applies to in the population as a whole is small. But what about the rest, the survivors? Where across the range of birthweights would we expect the chance of survival to be greatest? Wouldn't we expect it to be around the average birthweight, as this is the most common birthweight in the population? Wouldn't babies right in the centre of the distribution of weights around birth be the most normal, and so the safest?

The answers to these questions are at first sight surprising. It turns out that the safest place on the graph to be born is at a substantially higher birthweight than that for the majority of babies. But this 'safe weight' applies to fewer than about 20% of the babies overall. Perhaps the better growth of these fetuses, perhaps having more body fat at birth, promoted their greater chance of survival – we don't know. What this safest weight is, will depend on the population studied.

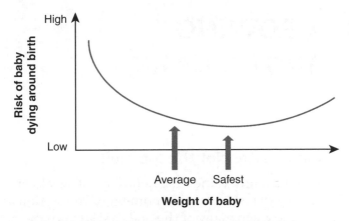

Figure 2.6 What is the safest birthweight at which to be born? Data from the Netherlands suggest that the safest weight is not the average birthweight for the population. It is substantially higher – around a weight achieved by fewer than 20% of babies.
Data from Vasak et al. 2015.

But the point is that for the majority of babies, even in this normal healthy Dutch population, birthweight is below the 'safest' weight. Even in the majority of babies, born with a birthweight around average, their fetal growth has been constrained. Their growth may have been less than ideal for fetal and neonatal survival. But it would be safer for their mothers in terms of delivery.

So most babies born today, and presumably throughout our history, are a bit smaller than they might have been, through the operation of maternal constraint of their growth.

Birth is seen as perhaps one of the most important milestones for parents – a time when a hidden tiny person is now visible to us all, and we can see that a new life is just beginning. In reality of course that new life started months earlier. Birth is an important transition, but is only a station on the journey.

We need to go back again in our story, to find out about the fetal phase of our lives.

3 GROWING IN THE DARK

The Stations Are Not the Journey

In our lifelong journey, the first 1,000 days of development is the first leg that starts at the moment of conception and ends at a time when many of the body's systems have gone through their most important period of development, at about two years of age. Journeys have milestones, like stations on a railway line. They mark our progress. The most helpful milestones are clear and unmissable, so that they can be seen even in the dark or in bad weather.

But passing milestones doesn't tell us anything about the nature of the journey itself. The stations on a train journey don't relate to how pleasant and smooth travelling was, for example the time spent delayed between stations, the lack of a seat or refreshment, the heating or air conditioning not working, and so on.

In just the same way, there are very clear and well-established markers of human development on that first leg of our life journey – and in the previous chapters we've referred to a few of the big ones, like being born, your first word, toilet training …

The big milestones in development are visible moments, but they should not be allowed to stand in for our attention to what is going on behind the scenes

These events are important milestones, but it is essential not to see them as development itself. They can loom as huge barriers which somehow have to be overcome, and families, peer groups and even health professionals can over-emphasise their importance. The big milestones are visible moments, but they should not be allowed to stand in for our attention to what is going on behind the scenes – the journey that's taking place between the stations.

The fetus has not just been waiting patiently to arrive at the destination of birth. It has been actively involved in the journey

---

This does not mean that they should be viewed merely as a box-ticking exercise which has no real relation to the ongoing process of development. They are more than that, especially if they flag up some serious problems. But it is the process of development which matters. The fetus has not just been waiting patiently to arrive at the destination of birth. It has been actively involved in the journey.

Many of the milestones of development are passed out of sight, and some have been visualised only relatively recently with new technological advances. In fact it has taken some visionary and sometimes contentious research to get to this point. A case in point is the controversy over the suggestion by the German doctor Johann Friedrich Ahlfeld that the fetus makes breathing movements in the womb.

Hold Your Breath

Johann Friedrich Ahlfeld's fellow doctors were getting fed up with him. Just because he was director of the prestigious women's clinic and school for midwives in Marburg, Germany, did not give him the right to keep insisting that they hear about his obsession. This was the late nineteenth century after all, and medicine was moving from guesswork and superstition to practice based on scientific evidence. Ahlfeld's ideas seemed

to be based on not much more than anecdotes or conversations with patients, not on rigorous investigation,
and so they seemed terribly out of date.

Ahlfeld was struck by the fact that every pregnant
woman reported feeling movements of her fetus in the
womb. But he was convinced that there was much more
to these than just random movements of the arms and
legs. He thought that, if carefully observed, they might
reveal that the fetus was making *breathing* movements.
His colleagues scoffed. How could the fetus be breathing, living as it did completely enclosed in amniotic fluid? Surely, everyone knew that babies start to breathe
after they are born.

Ahlfeld's idea was based on observations and reports
from pregnant women themselves. He listened to these
movements with a simple stethoscope-like device, and
repeatedly heard rapid, shallow movements of the fetal chest which he was sure were like breathing. But
his colleagues maintained that Ahlfeld's 'fetal breathing movements' must just be artefacts produced by the
mother's body or movements of her intestines.

Ahlfeld died in 1929, so he almost certainly did not
know of the work of Joseph Barcroft in Cambridge,
who tested his idea. Barcroft reported in 1930 that the
sheep fetus did indeed make rapid, shallow breathing
movements in the ewe's womb about a month into her
pregnancy. These were not breathing in the sense of
sucking air into the lungs, but breathing efforts nonetheless. The diaphragm, a sheet of muscle lying under
the lungs, was shown to contract and there were pressure changes in the trachea (the windpipe).

It wasn't until 1970 that researchers working sim-
ultaneously in Paris and Oxford showed beyond doubt
that the fetal sheep continued to make these breathing
movements in the womb until a day or so before birth.

And it was only with the new techniques of medical ultrasound, developed initially after the Second World War from modified ex-military instruments used to detect submarines, that the imaging of the human fetus revealed that it too was making these breathing movements in the womb.

Ahlfeld had been right all along.

Fetal movements are usually felt by the mother between 16 and 24 weeks of pregnancy. This is the so-called 'quickening' of the fetus. They might be gentle shifts in position, rather like a sleeper turning over in bed. They might also be quite forceful, like a kick or stretching a leg against the wall of the womb. The movements are small at first, and become stronger as the baby grows. In the days before pregnancy tests were available, it was these first movements which signalled to the woman that she really was pregnant.

Feeling these movements confirms that the baby is alive, and this has been a source of relief for many parents for generations. King Henry VIII (1491–1547) was desperate to have a male heir to succeed him on the throne of England, so when his third queen, Jane Seymour, reported feeling the quickening of a baby in her womb, money was distributed for Londoners to celebrate on free wine, and the bells of St. Paul's Cathedral were rung.

Quickening was a milestone in pregnancy, and one that had already influenced medieval (around fifth to thirteenth century) laws in many European countries, that an abortion produced in a woman by poison or physical violence did not count as murder of her baby until after the quickening. Even Aristotle (384–322 BCE) wrote about quickening, although it is true that he said, with less accuracy, that male fetuses take on human characteristics such as moving about after 40 days in the womb, and female fetuses not until about 80 days.

To Sleep, Perchance to Dream

The studies on fetal breathing movements, started by von Ahlfeld, opened up the question of the origins of fetal behaviour, and so of course the function of our brains before birth. Like many organs in the fetal body, the brain starts to develop in the first three months of pregnancy, but it isn't until the next three months that its function really starts to be felt. At this time the fetus is starting to make body movements and so the neural wiring to carry these out must have formed, even if the movements are not under the conscious control of the fetus.

As with its breathing movements, there seems to be a pattern to these body movements. They don't occur all the time, and are particularly noticeable in the evening after the mother has eaten. With modern ultrasound scanning techniques, we can watch these movements in detail. Because the fetus is suspended in its amniotic fluid in the womb, the movements in the early stages of pregnancy can appear much more smooth and graceful than they will be soon after the baby is born. They are more like underwater movements in a swimming pool.

The fetus often touches its face, sometimes sucks a thumb or fingers, stretches its limbs and yawns. Is it boring living in the womb? Its eyes move about rapidly. Later in pregnancy the fetus is more cramped and so its movements are more limited in scope, but it has very strong muscles. It can be startled by a loud noise, shooting its arms and legs out and making its presence very definitely felt by its mother.

Watching these activities before birth on the screen of an ultrasound machine is fascinating and of course for parents it gives the first real movie clip of their baby. But although ultrasound is very safe in clinical use, it can't be used to watch fetal behaviour for more than short periods of time.

Researchers have however been able to watch for longer periods in some large animals such as sheep, where many aspects of fetal development are similar to our own. In these studies, it has even been possible to make recordings of the fetal EEG (electroencephalogram), the brainwaves which are used in some human psychological studies or in a lie detector, and in studies of sleep and behaviour.

As adults, when we fall asleep, characteristic patterns of these brain waves appear. In one sleep state, large waves of EEG electrical activity occur and at this time we usually lie quietly and breathe regularly. After a while, another pattern appears. The activity becomes more erratic with a pattern of many small rapid electrical waves. We now breathe irregularly and we make random body and limb movements, ranging from twitches to quite forceful actions. If we watch someone who is asleep at this time, we can see that their eyes move around rapidly too, in little bursts, even though their eyelids remain closed. We can observe something similar in a dog or a cat, happily asleep in their basket or on the hearthrug.

We know that this second pattern of activity is associated with dreaming, and it appears to be essential to the functioning of our brains. Dreaming may help us to make sense of our experiences when we are awake, and allow the brain to organise itself. Children show this pattern of rapid eye movements or 'active' sleep, alternating with periods of 'quiet' sleep, and it appears to be necessary for their brain development. The sheep fetus shows these sleep state patterns in the womb from mid-gestation with a quiet pattern alternating with periods of jerky movements, rapid movement of the eyes and breathing.

But even during these active periods it seems that the brain connections aren't all in place. If the fetus is ever 'conscious' – and this is debatable – then it would only seem to be so for brief episodes. Reaction to touch, smell and sound must operate at an unconscious level. These active episodes of the fetus can last a few minutes, and then the fetus appears to pass into quiet sleep – not moving, often not 'breathing', and with only slow movements of the eyes.

So do we dream when we are in the womb? From the patterns of body, breathing and eye movements, so similar to those in our adult dreaming sleep, we would have to say that it seems that we do. But what on earth can a fetus be dreaming about? We have no idea, although we can say that, just as after birth, dreaming and the periods of active and quiet sleep are probably necessary activities for brain development and function.

Although there are extended periods when newborn babies are asleep, when they are awake they often make their presence felt. Their demands for food, warmth and comfort are very apparent to anyone within earshot. Being awake is associated with a very excitable pattern of EEG activity, not surprising because the brain is being flooded with sensory information and is producing a range of activities. So perhaps we shouldn't be surprised that the fetal brainwaves show some short patterns in later gestation which seem to resemble an excitable wakefulness pattern that does not seem to be either quiet or active sleep.

Be Prepared

The more important an event is, the more important it is to be prepared for it, and to rehearse – to have a 'dry run'. It might be rehearsing the flow of a marriage or partnership ceremony, or a speech after dinner to your guests, which can be nerve-wracking if you aren't used to public speaking. Or perhaps, if you are going for an important job interview next Monday, it's not a bad idea

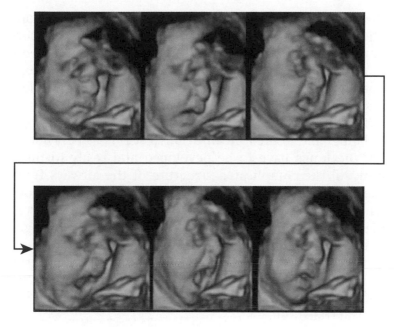

Figure 3.1 Is it boring in the womb? The fetus is caught before, during and after a yawn using three-dimensional ultrasound imaging. The purpose and function of the yawn is uncertain but is part of normal fetal development.

N Reissland Durham University.

to spend some time over the weekend thinking about what questions you may be asked and rehearsing your answers.

A dancer won't only work for months to perfect a routine for a performance, but even before rehearsals they'll warm up, to get their system ready.

In the previous chapter we saw how dangerous the process, the simple mechanics, of being born can be. But the challenge does not stop there. As soon as the baby is born, its vital supply of oxygenated and nutritious blood, through the umbilical cord from the placenta, is cut off. The baby has to start to breathe air. This is vitally important and it can't afford to mess this up. It makes sense to rehearse it in advance. It's rather analogous to the old Russian proverb useful to many a carpenter or tailor: 'measure seven times, cut once'.

The more we think about it, the greater the challenge of being able to breathe air at birth seems to be. First of all, the lungs have to be developed and ready to function. All the complicated structure of the airways from the windpipe down to the tiny alveoli, the air sacs across which transfer of oxygen and carbon dioxide (CO_2) takes place, have to be ready. This happens gradually throughout pregnancy, but the final preparations are made only in the last few weeks. This is why babies born preterm sometimes have trouble breathing, as they did not have enough time in the womb to prepare their lungs for this critical transition.

Researchers following the lead of Ahlfeld and then Barcroft have now shown that the fetus starts to make breathing movements early in gestation

---

Researchers following the lead of von Ahlfeld and then Barcroft have now shown that the fetus starts to make breathing movements early in gestation, although they are very rapid and shallow. Inside the womb, fluid in the baby's lungs is secreted continuously by them and this then passes out through the fetal mouth into the amniotic cavity. The fetus does not inhale the amniotic fluid that surrounds it. The fetal breathing movements do not pull fluid back into its lungs but they help to develop the diaphragm and the muscles attached to the ribs that will be used to breathe air for its entire life after birth. The breathing also distorts the airways and the alveoli, which stimulates them to develop.

Practice Makes Perfect

So starting to make breathing movements after birth should not be difficult, because the fetus has been practising them for months.

The real challenge is getting rid of the fluid which fills its lungs, so that they can be inflated with air: otherwise the body will literally drown itself. In the past, a midwife or the person helping to deliver the baby might hold it by the ankles, upside down, and swing it gently to and fro in the hope of draining the fluid from the lungs.

This was a nice idea, but is completely ineffective. The fluid fills all the tiny alveoli, so the baby has to get rid of this liquid in its lungs itself. How does it do this? By crying? No, because not all newborn babies cry and it isn't easy to see how this would empty the lungs.

The baby has to take fluid back up from the lungs into the bloodstream and reduce the production of any more fluid. This movement of fluid into or out of the lung is controlled by tiny chemical pumps in the walls of the lung cells. These pumps move the components of salt – sodium or chlorine – in one direction or the other and water follows them. So when, within a matter of minutes of being born, liquid stops being secreted into the lungs and is instead taken back into the bloodstream, it is because these pumps have changed direction. The trigger for this change in fluid direction comes from a set of hormonal changes in the baby's bloodstream which happen at birth.

Have a Heart

Filling the lungs with air at birth is vital but it will only keep the baby alive if the oxygen in the air can be transported around the rest of the body. So by birth, the lungs need a good supply of blood that will take up oxygen and deliver it to where it is needed for use by cell metabolism around the body. This metabolism produces CO_2 and the blood circulating in our bodies delivers this CO_2 back to the lungs so that it can excreted.

Before birth, the fetal lungs aren't doing this. They have a supply of blood, but only enough to grow them; the picking up of oxygen or getting rid of fetal CO_2 is done by the placenta rather than the lungs. Then, at birth, suddenly the flow of blood to the lungs has to pick up enough oxygen to keep the entire body alive. This requires some substantial and speedy re-arrangements of the plumbing of the fetal circulation.

Consider your heart for a moment. The chambers on the right side of the heart – the right atrium and ventricle – receive blood returning from the body in the veins and pump it to the lungs to pick up oxygen and get rid of CO_2. The left side of the heart – the left atrium and ventricle – receives that oxygenated blood returning from the lungs and then pumps it to the body.

But before birth, the two sides of the fetal heart work together in parallel. They pump only a little blood to the lungs to keep them growing and all the rest to the fetal body and also to the placenta. This is essential because it's the placenta which is keeping the fetus alive and growing, taking on not only the roles of the lungs but also the kidneys and the intestines.

This fetal plumbing is a temporary fix. It works firstly because there is an opening between the right and left sides of the heart, so not all the blood returning from the body has to go to the lungs. Secondly, there is a bypass or shunt in the blood vessel plumbing so that not all blood pumped out by the right side of the heart before birth has to go to the lungs. The 'hole in the heart' and the blood vessel shunt close up after birth through a combination of mechanical processes as the lungs inflate and changes in local and blood-borne chemical signals.

The hole between the two sides of the heart will close naturally after birth, but if it does not the baby will not be able to pump enough oxygenated blood to the body, and will look 'blue'. This condition was fatal until pioneering surgical methods were developed in the middle of the twentieth century to close the hole. They required developing a heart–lung machine, which could take over its work while the surgeon operated on the baby's heart to close the hole. Today such procedures are routine and the chances of survival of the baby, and the subsequent perfectly healthy life of the child, are very high.

The fetal heart is one of the first organs to develop. In the embryo, the heart starts to beat about three weeks after fertilisation. This is a point at which the embryo is becoming almost too big to obtain the oxygen and the nutrients it needs just by diffusion from the fluid surrounding it in the womb. It needs its own internal transport system, the circulation of blood driven by the heart.

As the fetus grows, so too the veins and arteries of the fetal circulation grow, and the heart grows in size and strength accordingly, increasing the number of its muscle cells by cell division to meet the demands placed on it. Then, in the last few weeks of gestation, the heart's cells stop dividing, effectively never to do so again. This is a little surprising, because it means that at birth we have the full number of heart muscle cells that will have to last us for the rest of our lives.

The heart will beat on average more than two billion times during our lives, but its muscle cells can never take a break ... heart cells we've grown before birth have to last us a lifetime

---

The heart will beat on average more than two billion times during the course of our lives, but its muscle cells can never pass the job on to new ones or take a break. Of course the heart cells aren't all working at maximum power all the time, and it may be that some stem cells can develop into a few new heart muscle cells if needed. But effectively, that's it. The heart cells we've grown before birth have to last us for a lifetime. And for a life about which the fetus at birth can have no idea.

How big will the person that this heart needs to serve, be? How physically active will they be? How long will they live? It seems to us as scientists that developing the heart like this is a very risky investment gamble for the fetus to make without some 'insider information' about the life it will lead and what it will need. More about this in a moment.

Water Baby

Imagine the fetus sitting in a sea of its own urine. Nice thought, isn't it?

Some people maintain that soaking your feet in your own urine can soften the skin and fight infection. Imagine then, the fetus sitting in a sea of its own urine. Nice thought, isn't it?

The fetal kidneys are formed by mid-gestation and work from the outset to get rid of waste products that come from cells when they do what they do best – grow, divide, make structural proteins, hormones etc. This waste is passed out as dilute urine into the amniotic cavity which surrounds the fetus. Usually there is no shortage of water for the fetus, which can take up as much as it needs from the mother across the placenta.

It is only after birth that we need to be more careful and to conserve body water. So we have to control the amount of water to be passed out in the urine, and this is one of the tasks of the kidneys. After birth, as blood passes through them, the kidneys take more water back up into the body than they did during fetal life and so they make more concentrated urine.

Life wouldn't be easy if we passed 175 litres of urine a day – we would spend our lives in toilets and drinking water. The strange way our kidneys work arose way back in the mists of evolutionary past, because the species from which we evolved lived in the sea

---

We have about a million filtering units (nephrons) in each of our two kidneys, which together typically filter the complete volume of our blood, which is about 5 litres in adults, about 35 times every day. Most of this water is reabsorbed into the body, which means we don't usually pass more than about 1.0–1.5 litres of urine each day. Life wouldn't be easy if we passed all the urine the kidneys make before reabsorbing most of the water. That's about 175 litres of urine a day – we would spend our lives in toilets and drinking water.

The strange way our kidneys work arose way back in the mists of evolutionary past. The species from which we evolved lived in the sea. As aquatic beings, getting rid of water absorbed was the goal, so kidneys were developed which extracted vast amounts of water from the bloodstream. It was only when our ancestors became land animals that keeping water in their bodies became the challenge and it was necessary to add another process to kidney function, to reabsorb nearly all of the filtered water.

The functions of the kidneys are controlled, according to how much water and salt we consume and the demands of our bodies to excrete the waste products of metabolism. Water retention is far more of a challenge if we are exercising hard in a desert than sitting quietly in a cool climate. In addition, what the kidneys do to control the amount of fluid in our bodies, and what's in that fluid, is a big part of how our blood pressure is kept within normal limits. As we age, the function of the kidney's nephrons declines.

So the more nephrons we had developed as fetuses, the longer we are likely to be able to sustain good kidney function, and so control of our blood pressure within healthy limits.

Investing in Our Bodies

Do you want to own your home or would you prefer to rent it? Renting has the advantage that you don't need to think too far ahead and it keeps you flexible, ready to move off again. If you invest in buying your own home you may lose some flexibility but, on the other hand it may increase in value, making your life more comfortable and secure later. Develop the right strategy at the right time and it can pay rewards in the long term. Get it wrong and it can be a costly mistake with long-term consequences.

The investment we made in developing some parts of our bodies before we were born is effectively permanent. Some organs, such as our skin and our intestines, are continually being renewed, so we have to devote resources to them all our lives. But for others, such as our hearts and kidneys, the one-off investment we made during our development is irreversible. We have to live with the consequences. We can't move to another body in the way that we might move house.

Could it be that the fetus has decided how many of each of these crucial heart and kidney cells to develop, 'anticipating' somehow that this will be a reasonably good prediction of the numbers that the person will need later? Why not just develop a good supply plus a few thousands spare?

The answer is the same as for buying a home. If you opt for one for which you can't afford to pay the mortgage, one that has more rooms that you really need and that uses up money you don't have in heating and services, then you may not have made a smart move and your future financial stability may be at risk. In a similar way, developing the body before birth uses nutrition which isn't always in plentiful supply. And once developed each of these heart muscle cells and nephrons will need to be maintained for the rest of our lives, using up vital nutrients and oxygen. The kidneys and the heart are expensive organs to run – for example, in our adult lives about one quarter of the blood pumped out by our hearts every minute supplies our kidneys.

And so it appears that the fetus develops an appropriate number of these kidney nephrons and heart cells on an individual basis, based on signals it receives about the world outside – we have customised hearts and kidneys.

Some of the signals that allow this specific kidney and heart development for each of us may come from the genes we inherit from our parents, which they inherited from their parents in turn, and so on back over many generations. Those genes will have been selected and tuned in terms of what best fits the environment in which we live.

Recent research has revealed that important signals pass to the fetus across the placenta, telling it about the mother's nutrition, proportions of fat, muscle and bone, heart function, blood vessels, kidneys and her lifestyle

---

But research in recent decades has revealed that much more important signals pass to the fetus across the placenta, telling it about the mother's nutrition, her body composition (her proportions of fat, muscle and bone), the function of her heart, blood vessels and kidneys and about her lifestyle. Such signals are specific to that pregnancy. They are likely to be the best signals for the fetus to use, because they are probably likely to reflect the environment into which a particular baby will be born. We'll come back to the question of what happens if that prediction is wrong in Chapter 5.

There are several other organs of the body which the fetus must develop to be ready to start independent life after birth, even though they are not needed for growth or survival prenatally. A good example is the gut. The fetal gut will be exposed to amniotic fluid that is swallowed, and the gut can produce a small amount of faeces, especially near birth.

The gut isn't providing nutrition to the body until the newborn baby's first feed. But gut development in the fetus during pregnancy can be compromised if it isn't getting sufficient nutrition or oxygen across the placenta, and this problem will become apparent only after birth when for the first time it needs to do digestion work.

Another example relates to body fat. The vast majority of the fat storing cells, called adipocytes, in our bodies are formed in our fetal life too. Depending on the food we eat and the physical activity we take, they are called upon to store more or less fat throughout our lives. So they can expand or contract, but their numbers don't change. But as with heart muscle cells and kidney nephrons, it seems that we forecast how many fat cells we are likely to need before birth, before we actually need to use them to full capacity.

Similar considerations apply to the cells that make up the fibres in our skeletal muscles. Different muscles have properties which affect how they contract – the large muscles in our legs are able to contract fast so that we can make rapid movements, whereas those in our backs are better suited to the slow, steady contractions we need to maintain posture. We might be able to top-up damaged fibres from some precursor cells present in adult muscle, but the broad number and type of muscle fibres seems to be set before birth.

Muscle isn't just important for our mobility and posture, though. Like fat, it plays an important role in the control of our metabolism, especially how our bodies use glucose. So perhaps the fetus forecasting its need for muscle before birth will be helpful in protecting it from diseases like diabetes. In people with a form of diabetes known as Type-2 Diabetes Mellitus, their skeletal muscles are less able to help in taking up glucose after a meal.

There are other tissues which can be replenished throughout our lives – such as skin, bones and blood cells. Because these have to be renewed it seems that the fetus could not make any useful predictions about our later needs. In any case it would be impossible to be equipped at birth with all the blood cells that we'll need for our lives as the average lifespan of the red blood cells in our bloodstream is only about 120 days. We have to make new ones all the time.

One of the major themes of this book is control. It is quite startling to realise how little control over our destiny we have as adults

One of the major themes of this book is control. It is quite startling to realise how little control over our destiny we have as adults. From what we have revealed in this chapter, we make investments into much of what controls us, how our bodies work and our future health or risk of disease, early on in our lives. We've placed our bets on the outcome of our future, and have to live with the consequences.

We are developing in the dark and we don't remember anything about it.

A Taste of the Future

The mothers and fathers of unborn children have probably always speculated on what the effect of the mother's life on her fetus might be. Would eating broccoli in pregnancy mean that the child would be different from most others in gobbling up their greens? Or, returning to the risks of obstructed labour which we discussed earlier, would avoiding drinking milk help to keep the fetus small and reduce the chance of this dangerous event?

There is now considerable evidence that the fetus can respond and adapt to cues from the mother's environment. This is a very important discovery

---

In the main, scientific research has not found any evidence for such myths or superstitions. But despite that, there is now considerable evidence that the fetus can respond and adapt to cues from the mother's environment. This is a very important discovery.

There are critical elements of the mother's diet which are essential for healthy fetal development. The most obvious is folic acid, because women who don't take the recommended supplement of 400 micrograms a day (before pregnancy and for the first 12 weeks of pregnancy) have an increased risk of their baby developing spina bifida. The fetus exposed to excessive levels of blood glucose because the mother has developed gestational diabetes may grow too large for easy delivery, making early diagnosis and treatment of the condition very important. And much ongoing research concerns components of the mother's diet such as oily fish as a supply of the fatty acids important to development of many fetal organs.

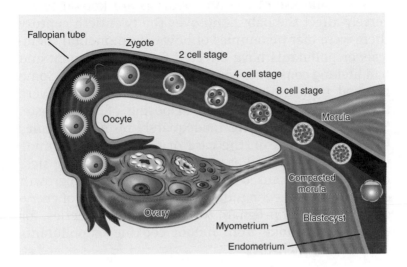

Figure 3.2 The early embryo in the Fallopian tube It takes several days before the fertilised egg implants into the lining of the mother's womb. Even before the placenta forms, it's receiving signals from the fluid in the Fallopian tube about the environment into which it will eventually be born. The way in which it adapts to those cues can influence how it will respond to the world after birth.

The unborn baby, even when just a newly fertilised egg (embryo) can sense aspects of the mother's diet, such as glucose or amino acids or fats. Recent research shows that these cues can affect the way cells in different parts of the embryo or fetal body grow, directly, by altering how the DNA of the inherited genes works. This is a process known as epigenetics. But these cues from the mother's world can also change the flow of blood around the unborn baby's body to prioritise blood flow to the most important organs, like the heart.

Although no-one now believes that a mother frightened by a bull in late pregnancy will deliver a baby with bovine features, aspects of maternal behaviour such as smoking and use of alcohol or drugs are known to adversely affect the baby. And over the twentieth century there were many examples of how environmental chemicals or pollutants have affected fetal development and had lifelong consequences for the next generation. Some resulted from industrial chemical spillage, some were the results of negligence in disposing of toxic waste. Some were from taking inadequately tested medicines in pregnancy, like in the case of the drug thalidomide which was prescribed as a treatment for morning sickness, but which caused abnormalities in the fetal growth of the limbs. But even today some are the result of everyday exposures of pregnant women in some societies, for example, to smoke from indoor cooking or pollutants from nearby highways.

Nobody Is Perfect

This new science which shows that the fetus can adapt to early influences from the mother's environment, her nutrition, body composition and lifestyle, starts to make sense of the seemingly endless variation that we see in human beings. We are all different and we all have different bodies. Ever since Charles Darwin published his theory of evolution in 1859, we have been aware that the differences between the members of a species – our own species included – are important for how the range of life that exists on our planet came to be. Not everyone agreed with Darwin then, and some people still disagree with the fundamental concept of evolution today, but no-one can deny that variation exists.

Variation is a good thing ... because if we all have the same characteristics and the same vulnerabilities, then a single challenge could wipe out everyone

We're each individual, and nobody is perfect. Variation is a good thing. At the very least, life would be very predictable and very dull without it. Every species needs variation in the characteristics of its individual members – because if we all have the same characteristics and the same vulnerabilities, then a single challenge could wipe out everyone. So survival and continued evolution depend on the insurance which variation provides against challenges.

We don't know what those challenges might be in the future. What will our environments be like and what will our bodies have to cope with? Just look at how worried most of us are about the effects of climate change, or fast food or social media, on our lives. A generation ago, these problems were not a concern to any of us. We did not worry about them because we did not know about them.

It is shocking how fast such unanticipated problems can arise. Some scientists think that we are living in a new period of the Earth's history – the so-called Anthropocene – where human activities have changed the nature of our planet, possibly for ever. It is certainly true that some of the changes which we have produced are irreversible.

By the time you read this it is almost certain that there will be no white rhinos left on the Earth: there are only two now and they are both female. Their numbers have been reduced to extinction by hunting and poaching in the shrinking territory allowed for them. Perhaps we will become extinct too, like the dinosaurs in the Jurassic period which were unable to survive extreme environmental changes following a meteorite strike. Or maybe only some of us will survive – who knows?

We won't dwell on these depressing prospects further. But what is clear is that it's a good plan for any species to have some variation in characteristics, so that hopefully some members of the species will survive as a result of their particular characteristics. There is no way of knowing which variations in which particular characteristics will turn out to be beneficial, but some useful predictions can be made from past experience, even though there's always an element of chance involved. These predictions are important in influencing how we develop as individuals.

We can't predict everything, so being prepared with the 'perfect body' is just not feasible. A set of features or characteristics which may be useful today, which seem just perfect, may turn out to be highly disadvantageous tomorrow in an unpredictable world – for our health or just raw survival. We'll see some examples of this later in the book.

In the Darkroom

We are used to watching as our bodies in childhood or adult life get moulded by the world around us. These are the processes by which they detect aspects of the world in which we live, and what we are doing in that world, and respond accordingly.

Our skin weathers, muscles grow or shrink, our weight goes up or down and we learn new things and forget others.

Some of these changes go hand-in-hand with the processes of ageing, which are slow and which we can't alter much. But our bodies are changing all the time in response to our environments in imperceptible ways, which may be very subtle. We are continuously adapting.

The adaptations may be temporary, for example the physiological changes in our metabolism, how the blood pumped by our hearts is distributed about the body and how content we feel after we have eaten a meal. Or they may be more sustained and longer term, for example the changes in our muscles, heart and blood vessels which occur in response to the level of physical activity we undertake regularly.

How much should we really expect to be able to adapt or control our bodies as adults? Very few individuals can train successfully for an Iron Man event at any time in their lives. It requires some special characteristics of fitness and endurance, even before the training programme, which not many of us possess. And even something more modest, such as running a half-marathon, isn't usually feasible in elderly people if they haven't kept up an appropriate fitness schedule from their middle age at least.

This idea of adapting to the world lies at the heart of why we wrote this book. Our early development, the processes by which our bodies grow and work in the womb and during infancy, is the most important time for adapting, but we have no memory of it.

Much of the adaptation takes place behind the scenes, hidden and little understood until recently, but nevertheless it shapes the rest of our lives. New research and technologies have allowed us to see what's going on in this hidden phase of our lives – and some of it is really surprising. The facts discovered in this chapter, for example that the embryo and fetus can sense changes in the mother's nutrition and adapt growth of blood circulation systems and vital organs, have challenged recent medical thinking about the origins of common diseases. We have become increasingly aware that the processes of this development have very far-reaching consequences.

The average life expectancy for a woman in the UK today is just over 83 years – that's 1,000 months. So, 1,000 days for a 1,000 months? The effects of our development certainly have a long legacy

---

Our development matters enormously, not just when we are in the womb or as infants, but literally in shaping our bodies for the rest of our lives. It affects us individually in controlling our bodies in the environment in which we find ourselves. And it matters to the prospects for a long and healthy life which we want to pass on to the next generation. A colleague suggested that our ideas might be summarised in the phrase: '1,000 days for 1,000 months' because 1,000 months (83.3 years) is currently the time which the average female baby can expect to live in the UK right now. It makes it clear why investing in development has such a good return, but also why the effects of poor development have a long legacy.

Perhaps it is helpful to think of human development like film photography. In the days before digital cameras and smartphones, pictures taken on film stayed in the camera until all the frames had been used, and then photographers needed to lock themselves in a darkroom to process their photos. The film was taken out of the camera and loaded into a sealed container a bit like a cocktail shaker, to which chemicals were added.

After washing and drying, the process of developing a frame on the film into a paper print could begin. Light was focussed onto photographic paper through the film for a precise number of seconds, and then the paper was placed in a bath of 'developer', aptly named because this is the stage when the printed image develops. This stage could be done under red light, to which the paper isn't sensitive, allowing the photographer to see the image literally developing for the first time before their eyes. Chemicals would then be used to stop the development, to fix the print.

If the development process had been done well, the image should not change for the rest of its life. Photography museums still have some prints dating from the mid nineteenth century produced by the early pioneers of photography.

Photography using film meant that no-one could ever be certain how the image captured at the click of the camera's shutter would actually turn out in print. How it developed was partly a matter of chance, and partly under the control of the photographer. There were some rules about how to do the development, but also a range of possibilities for influencing the result before the image on the film on paper was fixed. The development process in the darkroom would be subtly different every time, and so every print produced would be slightly different.

The first nine months of our development, our embryonic and fetal life, does indeed occur in the dark, like developing a film. The result is hopefully a healthy newborn baby who grows to be a happy infant – crying or smiling, sleeping, feeding and defecating.

Such 'success', like a clear photographic print, might seem like a simple and straightforward biological process, like a chemical reaction. But this isn't correct. Development of the final photographic print depended far more on the photographer's experience and judgement than just the chemical reactions in the darkroom, and a lot of it involved preparatory work and learning the skills needed before a photo was even taken.

So too is human development influenced and controlled by a range of factors internal and external to the baby, making every person unique. And they start at the moment of conception, like clicking the shutter of the camera. That's when development starts.

And that brings us to the question of sex.

4 SEX APPEAL

Caught in the Act

Most of us don't like thinking much about our parents having sex. What were the circumstances of that act so fundamental to making us exist? We hardly like to think about it. It's a private matter.

Equally, we might find it rather amusing that scientists have spent time researching why we have sex. Isn't it obvious? Well in a way, yes. But then again maybe there is something more to find out here. After all, even though all living organisms propagate, to produce a new generation of individuals, they don't all do so through having sex. Or at least not sex as we know it.

Some bacteria can have a kind of sex where the genetic material from one bacterium is inserted into another. This changes the genes of a single parent, who may then go on to produce offspring asexually. Some plants, fungi and many microscopic forms of life can also reproduce asexually, for example by budding off a part of their bodies which then detaches to develop into another separate individual member of their species. And some organisms can reproduce sexually or asexually, depending on the circumstances.

The ability of some animals to switch between sexual and asexual reproduction may be quite surprising. Take for example the all-female population of stick insects which were recently discovered to be reproducing asexually on Tresco and some of the other islands of the Scilly Isles in the far south-west of England. The real surprise was that their near relatives were literally on the other side of the world in New Zealand, where some of them were breeding sexually and some not.

From an evolutionary point of view it might seem that asexual reproduction is not a very good strategy for a species. Without the mixing of different sets of genes which occurs through sex, a population might become too homogeneous in its characteristics and lack the defence which variation offers against extinction in the event of a major change in the environment. It seemed that the stick insects in Tresco had become isolated and so had changed into an asexually reproducing type of the species. But if so, why had they not become extinct? How long had they been living on Tresco and how did they get there?

The answer seems to lie with the special climate of the Scilly Isles. In their position off the west coast of England they get the benefit of the warm sea currents of the Gulfstream and so their climate is mild, even sub-tropical. In the early part of the twentieth century exotic plant collections were established on the islands, for example in the Tresco Abbey Gardens. Plants brought from New Zealand were established there, and it seems that they brought some stick insect visitors with them. Perhaps there were not enough males for a sexually reproducing colony to form and so eventually the females resorted to the alternative strategy of replicating asexually. Switching between the strategies has also been shown for some stick insect populations in New Zealand, so it seems to be part of its natural adaptive strategy

Fifty Shades of Variation

For humans as well as stick insects, having sex is the first step in creating variation between individuals in the population.

In the previous chapter, we noted that we differ from each other in many ways, both in what we are made of and how we'll respond to challenges to our health across the life course. Variation in the characteristics of the members of the species develops from the moment of fertilisation, and is fundamental to the concept of evolution, which was first put forward in Charles Darwin's famous book *The Origin of Species by Means of Natural Selection* published in 1859.

Darwin's book caused a storm of protest from those who saw it as heretical – they believed that the origin of all species, including humans, was only by divine creation. Darwin knew that he would be challenging this widely accepted 'creationist' view of life in English Victorian society, and was hesitant about publishing his ideas. It wasn't until he realised that a competitor, Alfred Russel Wallace, was about to publish a similar idea that he sent his book for publication. It took time for the far-reaching implications of Darwin's ideas to be realised. It's interesting that today the idea of evolution is associated inseparably with Darwin, but he only used the word 'evolved' once in *The Origin of Species* – the very last word on the last page.

The idea of evolution is associated inseparably with Darwin, but he only used the word 'evolved' once in The Origin of Species – on the last page

---

Three processes were essential to Darwin's idea of the origin of species: variation, selection and inheritance. Individuals with different characteristics have different chances of surviving for long enough to pass on their genes to their offspring. And different chances of being attractive to a possible mate. Over time, the variation in a particular characteristic between members of the species may change, because selection has filtered out those variants which were not successful reproducers. This in turn creates possibilities for new sets of characteristics in future members of the species, if they are selected by surviving long enough to breed. Ever so slowly, this could lead to new species evolving.

In most people's minds, sexual reproduction, the mixing up of genes from our parents, is what makes us different from one another. We don't know when the idea of mixing of characteristics through sex first became realised, but it was certainly known to the ancient Greeks, in particular in the writings of the philosopher Aristotle (384–322 BCE). He established many of the concepts, and even the methodology which underpins science as we think of it to this day. Aristotle is often credited with inventing science itself, especially the science of biology.

Aristotle argued that our understanding of life should be based on observation, not on dogma. And he wasn't afraid to tackle some very difficult questions, for example how the early embryo (the first stage of development until about 10 weeks of gestation) was given life, the trigger to grow to become a new person. Much of his work involved studying chick embryos, a method that is still used today and which has given many insights into the biology of development. Many of his ideas have stood the test of scientific investigation over time.

Some others have not.

Without the benefit of a microscope, Aristotle was not able to visualise the fertilisation event which precedes the formation of the embryo. He did know that sex was necessary, and he guessed that giving a new embryo life required the fusion of something male and something female, but he was rather confused about how this worked. The male part was obviously semen, but he was suitably contemptuous of the idea of his predecessor Anaxagoras who suggested that the semen from the right testicle produced boys and that from the left produced girls.

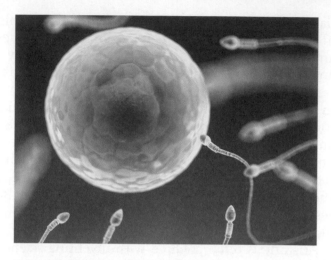

Figure 4.1 The moment of fertilisation Being able to see
fertilisation under the microscope has reshaped our
ability to control it, and is improving our understanding
of how conditions very early in our first 1,000 days affect
lifelong health.
SCIEPRO/Getty Images.

A convert to this idea, named Leophanes, suggested that
selecting the sex of children could be achieved by tying off
one testicle or the other. History does not record whether
he or anyone else tested this idea.

Aristotle thought that it was the foaming semen which
gave life to the embryo, and that the nourishment came
from the woman in the form of her menstrual blood. This
of course was completely incorrect. He suggested that if
the embryo was not enlivened enough by the semen, then
a female child would result – so his ideas became more and
more bizarre to our modern way of thinking.

When we look back at these ideas today, despite his insights into the scientific method, Aristotle does not come
off well. He was extremely sexist, probably like many
men of his day, believing that women were inferior, less

well-developed human beings than men. They were the product of an imperfect procreation process, he thought, in which not enough 'heat' was produced.

Amazingly, it wasn't until many centuries later that the details of fertilisation were finally discovered. The invention of microscopes in the seventeenth century wasn't enough on its own, because their lenses were not very good and scientific dogma influenced the interpretation of what was seen through them. It wasn't until 1875 that Oskar Hertwig showed beyond doubt that fertilisation involved the fusion of a sperm and an egg – albeit in the sea urchin where the eggs are bigger.

It wasn't until 1875 that Oskar Hertwig showed beyond doubt that fertilisation involved the fusion of a sperm and an egg

---

Coding

Sex is a highly effective way of creating variation between individuals, just so long as egg does manage to meet sperm. In the control centre, the nucleus, of most of the cells in our bodies we have 23 pairs of chromosomes (the exception being our red blood cells which don't have a nucleus and the sperm or eggs which have 23 single chromosomes). Chromosomes contain our DNA, arranged into patterns, or genes. For most cells, the pairs of chromosomes can be separated from each other.

The chromosomes have in total about 20,000–25,000 genes. These are made up of a series of nucleotide bases of which there are only four types, given the letters A, C, G and T, and they are arranged in groups of three to provide a code (the DNA code). The triplets are arranged so that, when part of the code is read, it will trigger the cell's machinery to make a specific part of a protein.

Each protein will then have some role in making the cells in the body work.

To achieve a particular result, such as coding for eye colour, the DNA coding for a specific gene will need to be at a specific position in the chromosome, and of a specific fundamental structure. Slightly different versions of specific genes will code for variations in a characteristic, for example for eye colour variations in the code will result in the individual having blue, green or brown eyes.

Egg and sperm are different from most of the other cells in our bodies. They only contain one of each pair of the 23 chromosomes. So once the egg and sperm fuse, the fertilised egg, now called a zygote, will have 23 pairs of chromosomes. However, one chromosome from each pair will have come from the mother and one from the father. So right away sex gives rise to variety in terms of the zygote's genetic makeup.

But if all that happened at the time when the eggs and sperm are formed in the ovaries and testes respectively was the splitting of the two chromosomes, so that each so-called 'germ cell' made two identical eggs or two identical sperm, then the range of variations produced by sexual reproduction would be limited.

What actually happens is that, as the chromosomes split, the DNA from them gets mixed up between the newly formed germ cells (a process called 'recombination'). And because this happens initially during the production phase of each egg and each sperm, every egg and every sperm that forms has a unique genetic makeup. Not only are they all different from each other, but the combination of DNA in each will never have been present in any human egg or sperm, ever. Statistically it will never occur again in a future egg or sperm either.

So this gives each of us the maximum possible variation in the genetic material coming from our mother and our father.

Mr Shandy's Clock

Tristram Shandy is the hero of Lawrence Sterne's satirical book of the same name. It's a weird, amusing but
puzzling book, and it's very long. It was published in
several volumes starting in 1759 and, while the title an-
nounces that it concerns *The Life and Opinions of Tristram
Shandy, Gentleman*, it only concerns a fraction of his life.

Tristram is obsessed by the idea that what happened
to him in his very early life had all sorts of consequences for him later. He did not of course think that this
was the result of inherited genes, because genes had
not been discovered then, but of accidents over which
he had no control. His problems started even at his
conception. At the very moment of what should have
been conjugal bliss, he learns that his mother asked
his father whether he had remembered to wind up the
clock. Tristram's problems started right at that inauspi-
cious moment.

His misfortunes became clear when he was born. To
his father's dismay, his nose was flattened against his
face. Sterne's satirical book refers to the phallic implications of the length of the nose, which seem to have been
the subject of bawdy jokes in the eighteenth century. So
not only did Tristram look ugly but it seemed to cast bad
omens on his later sex life.

We know now from scientific research that the size
and shape of our noses is partly genetic. Tristram inherited it from some ancestor somewhere along the
line. But lack of knowledge of genes and the science of
inheritance meant that Tristram focussed on the events
around his conception, because of his parents' actions,
not the genes that were passed to him by his parents.

The nose is one thing, but Tristram's parents can't
be expected to shoulder all the responsibility of how

Tristram turned out. We know now that there are several reasons why a purely genetic answer to the question of inheritance is wrong.

In fact, Tristram had unwittingly put his finger on some really important ideas, and in this chapter we explore the events around conception that can have life-long consequences for staying in control and staying healthy into older age.

Variety Is the Spice

What all this means is that each of us carries within our DNA almost limitless possibilities for combinations of the code which will make a person. Many of us are able to look at our parents and marvel at similarities and differences between us and them, and wonder how that came about. Did that trait 'skip a generation' or was it due to something else? The fictional character Tristram Shandy, is wrestling with just these kinds of thoughts, in our case study box.

The DNA of the fertilised egg (zygote) is drawn from all the DNA variants of its ancestors, over billions of years from the species from which humans evolved

---

Even though the egg came from a particular mother and the sperm from a particular father, the specific genetic makeup of the zygote is not just a mixture of that of its parents. Its particular blend of DNA is drawn from all the DNA variants of its ancestors, over hundreds of thousands of years, and even over millions of years from the species from which humans evolved.

We might even say billions of years, because life on Earth dates from about almost four billion years ago, with the simplest organisms like bacteria having the planet to themselves for the first two billion or so. These simple bacterial organisms were now composed of a single cell, but the crucial point is that the cell contained genetic material.

It is astounding to think that we must have evidence in our DNA of the genetic material shared so widely between simple organisms more than two billion years ago. The same goes for all species of animals and plants. It's a rather humbling thought. We should forget the idea that we as a species are special. We may think that we're the smartest – but then we would think that, wouldn't we? In fact, we're part of a huge invisible republic of shared information about life and the environment of the planet, which goes back billions of years. That's quite a database!

We're part of a huge invisible republic of shared information about life and the environment of the planet, which goes back billions of years

---

A further source of variation arises because accidents occur in the copying process of the DNA when the eggs and sperm are themselves made. Sometimes these copying errors are in the fine structure of the genes; and sometimes a particular gene is copied more than once, or not at all. These errors, multiple repeats or deletions, may or may not have consequences for what proteins will be made and so how cells in the body work. Some of these errors will be passed on to future generations, and others won't.

A good example is the HTT gene which is associated with Huntingdon's disease. The HTT gene provides instructions for making a protein called huntingtin. Although the exact function of this protein is unknown, it plays an important role in the function of nerve cells and is essential for normal brain development before birth. Huntingtin is found in many of the body's tissues, but has the highest levels of activity in the brain. Within cells, this protein may be involved in chemical signalling, transporting materials, binding to proteins and other structures, and protecting the cell from self-destruction.

One region of the HTT gene contains a particular DNA segment whereby three DNA building blocks (cytosine, adenine and guanine), known as a CAG trinucleotide repeat, appear multiple times in a row. Usually this CAG grouping is repeated about 10–35 times within the gene, so it is certain that we will inherit it even after the recombination processes we noted earlier. But if further copying happens, giving an individual perhaps more than 40 repeats of this short CAG code, their nervous system will make a longer version than normal of the protein huntingtin, and it will disrupt the way their neurons work, resulting in the development of Huntingdon's disease over time. The severity of the disease, and how fast it develops across an individual's life course, will depend on how many extra repeats of the short DNA CAG code that they possess.

Then there is yet another source of genetic variation.

At fertilisation, chromosomes from the mother and chromosomes from the father combine in the zygote. From then on, the embryo grows by cell division and each new cell will have a pair of each chromosome, of which one member is from the mother and the other from the father. As the genes are lined up in the pairs, for any characteristic there will be a gene for that characteristic in one chromosome from the mother and another in the other chromosome from the father. But as development proceeds usually only one of the pair of genes inherited is actually functional, so that either the mother's or the father's copy is switched off chemically while the other remains functional. The scientific term for this is 'imprinting', and this source of variation means that the developing offspring will have some active genes from the egg, some from the sperm.

Grain of Salt

In some ways this all seems mathematically satisfying; different combinations and ordering of code contribute to our species variation. But as we said in Chapter 3, the variation in characteristics between us as individuals is due to far more than just the genetic mixture established soon after fertilisation.

The baby in the womb senses and adapts to cues from the mother and the outside world and we explored some of the science behind this in Chapter 3. Development is plastic. An even more recent revelation is that this sort of adaptation to the environment starts from the very moment the embryo is formed at fertilisation.

The zygote responds to aspects of its environment, such as a lower level of dietary protein, higher levels of fat or folate (folic acid) availability. Researchers have studied the cells in the embryo that are destined to become the fetus and others which give rise to the placenta and have found that maternal diet can change the way these embryonic cells grow and what proteins they produce. They have been able to link this to long-term effects on the individual's behaviour, metabolism and cardiovascular health.

Fathers are not left out of the picture. A high-fat or low-protein diet, obesity or smoking have been shown to alter sperm structure, cause DNA damage and to be linked to changes in their offspring's metabolic and cardiovascular health

---

Fathers are not left out of the picture. A high-fat or low-protein diet, obesity or smoking have been shown to alter sperm structure, cause DNA damage and to be linked to changes in their offspring's metabolic and cardiovascular health.

So, to put it another way, as environment will shape the development of the embryo from the very start, there is everything to play for in its future. This is indeed the start of the individual's life course of responses, and resilience and risk, which we discussed in the previous chapter. From the moment of conception every new member of the human race starts adapting to its environment.

Fertilisation usually happens in the Fallopian tube (see Figure 3.2 in Chapter 3). The egg, smaller than a grain of salt, released from the mother's ovary must pass down this tube to reach the uterus. As it does so, the early stages of development take place as it divides into 2, 4, 8, 16 cells … and so on. It forms a ball of cells, called a morula, four days after fertilisation. By the time it enters the uterus, this ball of cells has become partly hollow, to form a mass of cells at one side and a thin rim surrounding the rest. This is the blastocyst. It now has to meet the challenge of implanting in the wall of the uterus. The inner cell mass will go on to form the embryo itself. The thin outer layer of cells will form the placenta. As it enters the womb it will find its way to the lining, where secretions from the glands in the walls provide it with nourishment.

This is a tricky time, because many embryos do not manage to implant into the wall of the womb. If they don't, they'll die. We don't know how many potential embryos fail to make it at this time, but probably three out of every four do not. Nor do we know why such an apparent waste happens. The processes affecting the life of the early embryo have evolved to be optimal in us and other mammals over millions of years. So there must be a good reason for the loss. Perhaps there is some incompatibility between the mother and embryo, or perhaps the embryo is not showing an ability to adapt sufficiently to its environment. This is an area of active research.

Soon after the embryo has attached itself to the wall of the uterus, the cells which will form the placenta begin to invade that wall. Placental function requires that the blood vessels of the fetus that will develop come into close contact with the mother's blood. This poses another risk, because the developing offspring is effectively a foreign invader – it possesses genetic material from another person, the father. Normally such invasion would invoke an intense immune response in the body. So the mother's immune response has to be supressed if the growing baby is not to be rejected. If this process is not sufficiently effective, the blood vessels supplying the placenta from the mother will not open up sufficiently. This will be bad for fetal growth, but it also has effects on the mother. Because the volume of her blood has increased and her heart is pumping hard, not opening up the vessels in the placenta enough may make her blood pressure too high. This condition, known as pre-eclampsia, can be very dangerous. If it continues it can threaten the life of both the baby and the mother.

Pre-eclampsia does not seem to happen in other mammals, but why it is peculiarly human is not known. Some researchers think that it may result from a fundamental incompatibility between the mother's and the father's make-up, because the risk can change with different partners.

First Conversation

The exchange of information between the mother and the embryo starts even before the embryo has made contact with the lining of the womb, and it can have very important consequences. The sex of the embryo is set from the moment of fertilisation, and so if it is necessary to stop the development of one sex over the other, this is a time at which this could be done at an early stage.

Does such sex selection really occur? It seems that it does, at least in some animals

---

Does such sex selection really occur? It seems that it does, at least in some animals. In some species of deer, if the food available to the population is scarce then it makes sense – from an evolutionary or population survival point of view – to increase the number of females in the herd. They are the smaller of the two sexes and less demanding of food, and future population numbers will be determined more by the number of females than males. So even though about the same number of male and female embryos will start life at fertilisation, it is possible to alter the sex ratio of the fawns which will develop and be born.

We don't know how the female deer (doe) communicates the state of the outside world, in terms of the availability of food or numbers of predators or competing species, to her embryos; it might be a stress hormone or the level of nutrients in her blood stream. But we can see why evolving a mechanism for such communication at this time could be very efficient. Something similar happens in some rodents, but not in us, as far as we know.

It is important that there is a degree of communication between the mother and her developing embryo for other reasons as well. This conversation will keep development on track and optimal. Unlike many small mammals, humans do not produce litters of many offspring. Also, we look after our offspring for a relatively long period of time, not only during pregnancy but in childhood.

Rat pups are weaned after three weeks of life and they are sexually mature not long after. But then they seldom live for longer than about 18 months. The field mouse may live only a few weeks after birth, long enough to grow to sexual maturity and mate, before it gets picked off by an owl or a kestrel, catches an infection, is killed by bad weather or starves. Their reproductive strategy seems to be 'live fast, die young', with the production of many offspring, most of which will die in the wild, partly because they don't have a long childhood of parental nurturing to help them survive.

Many species of fish seem to be even more negligent as parents, just depositing hundreds of eggs in the sea and then ignoring those that have been fertilised by the thousands of sperm which have also been deposited after their parents' brief mating.

For biologists interested in evolution, ever since the time of Darwin, the concept of 'fitness' has been fundamental. So-called 'Darwinian fitness' is basically the ability to survive to reproduce, so it's measured by the number of children or, better still, the number of grandchildren, which an individual has. This is how successful individuals in the population pass on the attributes that have made them successful to the next generation. The strategy for small mammals might be to produce large numbers of offspring, of which just enough will survive to pass on the parents' characteristics to the next generation.

When we think about the investment of resources which goes into developing a new human being to reproductive age, and the fact that we don't produce many children in our lives, we realise that our evolved strategy is very different.

Humans aim to ensure that the development of every offspring is as healthy and well adapted to their likely environment as possible. Pregnancy and child rearing are relatively long periods of the life course, so there is plenty of time for communication between the mother, or both parents and other members of the family, and the offspring.

We aim to live much longer than mice. And we don't think of the years after we have had children, when we aren't in the business of passing on our genes to the next generation, as being superfluous. In addition to passing on a selection of our genes, we aim to pass on as much in the way of survival skills as possible to our children, in the hope that they too will have long lives. We educate them about life as we know it, whether in terms of our own personal experiences, or what as a society we think is important. This is the role of parents, grandparents and other relatives, as well as forming the basis of the school curriculum. Within limits, the child will change, both mentally and physically, through processes of learning, of adapting to their environment.

Controlling Conception

The trouble with the randomness of the variation between us all, which is partly set up at the moment of conception, is that it's just that – it's random. As humans we have been unhappy about random, unpredictable events since the beginning of time. Imagine the challenge which unpredictability posed to our ancestors about 15,000 years ago when we changed our lifestyle from hunter–gatherers to settled communities starting to cultivate crops and keep livestock. Why was the harvest bad this year? What's wrong with these animals? Faced with these life-threatening uncertainties it's easy to see how questions of cause and effect would arise.

Trying to answer such 'why' questions may be linked to the origins of superstitions or religions, with ideas about gods who needed to be kept happy. Have we done something to offend the gods – are they angry and are they punishing us with these storms? If the gods want to punish us, maybe we have to punish ourselves by sacrificing some of our best livestock or even our children. This logic seemed to operate in some ancient cultures, such as the Aztecs and Maya, in which ritually sacrificed individuals including children were entombed with precious stones and gold and silver grave goods. Whether this worked to improve environmental conditions or defeat enemies is probably less important than the strength of belief that it would.

The whole scientific process is also based on asking 'why' questions. But, as with superstition, our need to answer them isn't just about curiosity about why things happen or how they work. It's about finding ways to control our world, our environment – to make it more predictable.

Looked at this way, it's not surprising that for centuries we might want to control something as important as sex, or the attributes of the next generation who are conceived as a result.

We don't know when it became common knowledge that pregnancy was the result of sex

We don't know when it became common knowledge that pregnancy was the result of sex. It's not obvious, when you think about it. After all, the majority of sexual encounters do not result in conception, and a high proportion of fertilised eggs do not implant in the wall of the womb to start pregnancy.

We do know though that early civilisations had some simple, and probably not very effective, contraceptives ranging from an Ancient Egyptian crocodile dung and sour milk paste inserted in the vagina as an acidic barrier to sperm, to European women in the middle ages being advised to cut off the testicles of a live weasel and wear them wrapped in goose skin to ward off pregnancy. Trying to control conception has probably been going on for millennia.

On the other hand, having several children may be essential when childhood mortality from disease is high, as it was until the early twentieth century even in developed countries.

Reproduction is also traditionally a very good way of making alliances between rival communities and even families, connections which may be enforced, as with arranged marriages in some cultures, or on the other hand very definitely discouraged. Shakespeare used the rivalry between two leading families in fourteenth-century Verona as the backdrop for his tragedy of Romeo and Juliet, the star-crossed lovers from those rival families.

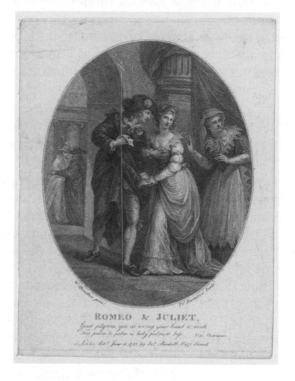

Figure 4.2 Romeo and Juliet No good will come from the liaison of the lovers from rival families.
The Metropolitan Museum of Art, New York, 17.3.1196, Harris Brisbane Dick Fund, 1917 www.metmuseum.org.

Most societies have a ruling class of high-status individuals, often in particular families such as nobility or royalty, with rules about the succession of wealth and power down generations. So it's essential to ensure that there are children to take over from their ruling class parents. The stakes can be high for conception when the sex of the offspring matters.

Henry VIII was so desperate to have a son as heir to the throne of England that he had two queens executed for being reproductively inadequate. It remains true that in many cultures today sons are far more valued than daughters, and there are many rituals and superstitions about how to conceive a boy rather than a girl. For example having sex under a full moon, in missionary position, facing a certain direction in bed, after drinking a prescribed potion or wearing a particular garment or trinket could result in conceiving a girl.

There are many rituals and superstitions about how to conceive a boy rather than a girl

---

From a purely biological point of view, as a species we produce slightly more boys than girls: 105 males for every 100 females are born in the UK each year. The reasons for this are not known, although it may simply be because the sperm with a Y chromosome, which will lead to a male embryo if it's successful in fertilising the egg, may be slightly lighter and able to swim just a little faster than its competitor with an X chromosome, which will lead to a female embryo.

However, until recently, the survival of boy babies was slightly less than that of girls, so the gender playing field started out fairly level. But there are data from some cultures which show substantially more boys being born, and more surviving, than girls. Is this because they have discovered a secret ingredient of sex to raise the chance of conceiving a boy?

No.

In some parts of the world small facilities operating outside hospitals offer ultrasound scans to pregnant women. Sometimes these facilities

advertise that they don't conduct fetal sex de-
termination. Unfortunately, the very mention of
the idea is a clue to what may go on

If you travel in some parts of the world, you'll see clinics offering ultrasound scans to pregnant women. These are often small facilities and operate outside hospitals, and they can provide a vital service to the community in terms of access to care in pregnancy. Sometimes, these clinics specifically advertise that they don't conduct fetal sex determination. Unfortunately, the very mention of the idea can give a clue to what may go on. It's not always possible to be certain of the sex of the fetus, but in a thorough scan to assess fetal growth and anatomy, placental attachment etc. it will usually be obvious if it's male. Another 'specialist', friend or family member may help with an attempted abortion if not. And there are reports of infanticide or very poor care of newborn girls, again sometimes by family members.

For over 40 years, China had an official programme to limit families to one child each. It was designed to control the growth of the population by making contraception widely available and enforcing it by financial incentives or sanctions, and even by forcing abortion or sterilisation. The policy achieved its aim of reducing population growth but having a girl was undesirable and drove increased practices of sex determination, abandonment and even infanticide. Reversal of the policy in light of economic pressures, low birth rates and an ageing population led the Chinese government in 2021 to allow all married couples to have up to three children.

Against this background of control, control of 'unwanted' baby girls or smaller population size, is the increasing demand for children in couples who find that they can't conceive. Infertility has always been a problem in our species, perhaps not surprisingly when we think of the low success rate between sex and pregnancy.

An added complication is infertility in men, sometimes due to sexual dysfunction. Henry VIII probably had diabetes associated with his severe obesity. As this is sometimes accompanied by erectile dysfunction it may have played a part in his problems in conceiving an heir. But sperm counts have been falling in men in Western countries over recent decades, and fewer sperm will inevitably lead to fewer conceptions. Pollutants in the environment may be partly to blame as they have been reported to produce changes in sperm structure.

Fertility in women is also falling, partly due to the fact that many women don't want to start a family until their thirties or older, to have more freedom and to establish a career. The availability of viable eggs in the ovary falls steadily during a woman's life and mathematical models predict that by the age of 30 she will only have 12% of the egg-producing follicles that she started life with left in her ovaries.

Technology to the Rescue

Such problems of course led to attempts to improve conception artificially. The earliest reports of artificial insemination were in animals during the late seventeenth and the eighteenth centuries. These came after the report in 1678 to The Royal Society of sperm seen under the microscope by Antoni van Leeuwenhoek and his assistant Johannes Ham in the Netherlands (we don't know whose sperm they were …).

The first documented case of artificial insemination in humans was from the physician John Hunter who helped a couple to conceive in London in the 1770s. These early attempts were largely concerned with the purely mechanical aspect of instilling the sperm into the vagina. But it wasn't until 200 years later that technology was developed

to perform fertilisation outside the woman's body altogether: Louise Brown, the first so-called 'test tube baby'
was born in Manchester in 1978. Patrick Steptoe and Rob-
erts Edwards, the scientist and doctor carrying out the
procedure, had mastered the technique of keeping the
fertilised embryo alive until it had matured to a ball of
eight cells, known as the morula, around three days after
in vitro fertilisation (IVF), before transferring it into the
mother's womb.

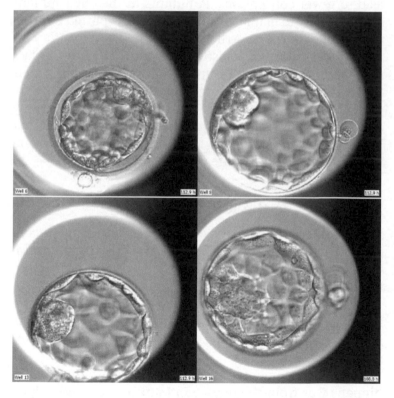

Figure 4.3 Embryos five days after artificial insemination Increasingly
sophisticated technologies help to select the embryo to implant which
will have the best chance of a successful pregnancy. Which one would
you choose?
TFP Wessex Fertility.

With the success of IVF, a new field of medicine and a new sphere of control over our lives was, literally, born. Now it became possible to help those couples who were having fertility problems because, with hormonal treatment, the woman could be induced to produce several eggs and healthy-looking sperm could be selected and injected directly into these eggs. Then the most healthy-looking embryos – sometimes several of them, although the number is strictly controlled in many countries – could be placed via a fine tube passed up into the womb.

But there were soon more possibilities available. As the embryo will develop normally even if one of its cells is removed at the stage when it has developed eight cells, now genetic testing could be carried out on one of its cells. The sex of the embryo could be discovered as could a range of severe inherited genetic conditions. Only the 'best' embryo(s) would be used.

The naturally occurring variation which Darwin had seen as essential to evolution, was now under our control

---

We had now invented control over one of the most fundamental processes of life – of evolution itself. The naturally occurring variation which Darwin had seen as essential to evolution was now under our control. So was the natural selection which he had envisaged as operating on this variation. The selection could hardly be less natural – occurring under the microscope and then in a Petri dish in a highly artificial environment, at the moment when the fertility specialist decided which embryo to implant and sucked it up into a tube.

The sperm and the eggs could also be stored. So now it became possible for a woman undergoing radiotherapy for cancer, which might induce genetic abnormalities in her eggs, to have some stored beforehand for IVF after the therapy had been conducted. An industry had been created. A sperm donor might be paid £150 for a sample of sperm which would sell for five times that to a woman wanting to conceive. Of course, if she wanted sperm from an identified donor – with just the 'right' attributes – the price might be much more.

Some couples and friends have helped one another in this difficult area of life – the start of its first 1,000 days. It has made same-sex parenting possible in new ways beyond adoption. And it has led to an industry in surrogate motherhood, commanding large sums of money and sometimes clandestine.

Liberating as the new ability to control reproduction has been, there remain many unanswered questions around IVF and all other forms of artificial reproductive technologies. It must be one of the most hotly debated areas of medicine. Ethical considerations go beyond the scope of this book. But some of the more scientific unknown implications of IVF are relevant. What are the possible lifelong effects of the undisclosed nutrient cocktail of the culture mediums in which the eggs are kept and the mechanical effects of handling the eggs and embryos in the procedures? Even though the methods are getting more sophisticated how should the 'best quality' embryo be decided?

These are all things that could influence the growth of the embryo in the very early stages and affect later health. In the USA 7.3 million women have received some form of medical care for fertility problems. There are ongoing studies following up babies born through artificial reproductive technologies into later life, but of course they will take many years to provide us with some answers. There are some reports that children born following IVF have a slightly higher risk of high blood pressure or risk factors for diabetes. Much more research is needed.

A relationships counsellor remarked that there are three things about which every couple will argue – sex, money and children. These three ingredients of trouble – or bliss – have from the 1970s been blended together in the laboratory into a cocktail to control the making of a person at the very start of their first 1,000 days.

The nuts and bolts, the technology behind actually making any type of artificial reproduction happen is considerable. And a big part of it is timing: for example, timing the collection of the mother's egg right in relation to the medication given to stimulate her eggs to mature, or to pick the optimum time to transfer the fertilised embryo into the mother's uterus.

When Is the Best Time to Be Conceived?

The events and their timing leading up to conception – whether natural or artificial – are crucial. This is the period of life which health professionals call the preconception period. Their conversations with couples undergoing fertility treatments focus especially on the behavioural and lifestyle issues which promote health in this period, with a view to promoting the best chance of a healthy pregnancy and having a healthy baby.

Much research has shown how having a poor diet, smoking, being obese, over-stressed or suffering domestic abuse can affect fertility and put the pregnancy at risk. Very recent research has shown that some of these factors can affect sperm quality too, and so they are issues for both men and women. But as so often, by far the greatest effects, and so the greatest burden of responsibility is laid at the feet of the woman. Getting ready for pregnancy in the preconception period seems to be more or less entirely down to her. You may not be surprised by this idea, but just because it is so widely believed does not mean that we should accept it uncritically.

But what actually *is* the preconception period?

From the perspective of the woman, preconception could be seen as the whole of reproductive life, from the time in her early teens when she started to menstruate to the menopause. But when we recall the hormone replacement treatments which are available and the regimes for inducing ovulation in preparation for IVF, it is clear that the end of reproductive capacity can be delayed.

The Guinness Book of Records tells us that the oldest woman to conceive 'naturally' in the UK was Dawn Brooke at the age of 59, but there are many other reports from around the world of older conceptions. Some used IVF like Daljinder Kaur who at 72 was believed to be oldest woman to give birth. With the use of donor eggs Maria del Carmen Bousada de Lara from Spain was over 66 when she became pregnant.

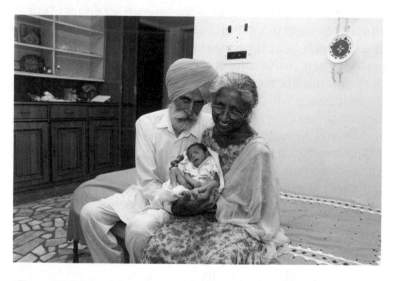

Figure 4.4 Age is no barrier to conception Technology makes it possible to conceive a baby at almost any age. Seventy-two-year-old mother Daljinder Kaur and husband, 79-year-old Mohinder Singh Gill, with their baby son Arman Singh on 11 May 2016, in Amritsar, India. Future Publishing/Getty Images.

The age at which menstruation starts, called menarche, is falling in most high-income countries, just as the age at which pregnancy is possible is increasing. This might be good news if it means that women's lives do not need to be totally focussed around the need to become mothers, as has often been the case throughout human history. But on the other hand, it might be felt that the new evidence on the importance of the mother's lifestyle and health in the preconception period means that girls' lives should be dominated by these concerns as soon as they enter their teenage years, and continue until middle age. This is a major responsibility. Is it equitable? Isn't it tough enough bearing children without having to take on this very long-term responsibility? Who is in control here?

On the one hand, new technologies give women more control, as the preconception period can be extended using technologies like IVF. But it is worth considering too that a woman's body changes with age – her shape, metabolism and more will affect her pregnancy. These are the sorts of things that make up 'maternal constraints' on fetal growth that we talked about in Chapter 3. We may have control over the preconception period, but when is the best time to be conceived?

There is also another way of looking at the issue. Without in any way diminishing the role of the mother (and her partner) in making choices about the timing and circumstances of possible conception, we could look at the situation from the point of view of the developing embryo and fetus. The most important aspect of our world before we were born was our mother's body – her diet, hormone levels, what she was doing and the function of her internal organs. Her body talked silently to ours, and we acted upon what she 'said'. We were 'listening' carefully. We only had one chance in life to form many of the vital organs in our bodies, so getting it right was really important. We live with the consequences for the rest of our lives.

If an embryo could choose when and how to be conceived, then what factors would it take into account?

Put like that, we might ask when is the best time to be conceived? If an embryo could choose when and how to be conceived, then what factors would it take into account? The mother's health, food availability, economic and social stability, infection, access to healthcare, levels of toxins and pollutants? The specific circumstances of conception can in various ways influence aspects of our future lives.

Most of these factors relate to the mother's life, and this reflects far more than just the circumstances of our parents having sex – the point at which we started this chapter. We can't go much further with our story without going back further before conception, to think very hard about wider societal issues affecting women's lives.

5 SHIT HAPPENS

Managing Expectations

Each of us can change from the moment of conception in response to signals from our mother's environment. Making a person is more than just their inherited genetic makeup. The embryo (and then the fetus) senses, in real time, the world around it – gauging the features of the world into which it will be born.

But is it enough? Shit happens, the world changes over time. The best laid plans turn out to be inadequate.

The developing embryo and fetus can't know what to expect, such as how many children their parents will have and so the competition for resources. Nor can they know the places where they will live over their life course. They can't predict how the world around will change as a result of human error, natural or man-made disasters or societal constructs.

So are any of the changes the developing embryo and fetus make from inside the womb going to be relevant to life outside the womb?

What might you ask if someone suggests that you consider living in a particular place in the world? The most obvious thing to ask is how safe that place is. There might be statistics about crime which you would want to know, but even before that you might ask about life expectancy there. How long, on average, do women and men living at that place live? This gives you a good idea about the access to healthcare there, how polluted the environment is, how easy it is to obtain a healthy diet and opportunities to get physical exercise, as well as the risk of life-threatening events such as conflict or violent crime.

But now think about this differently, based on what we've discussed in this book so far. Look at this from the perspective of a woman and her children, both before birth and in the world they are born into and inhabit for life.

Lives on the Line

The phrase 'the population explosion' was used commonly in the twentieth century to describe the concern that as a species we might reproduce to increase our numbers beyond the capacity which our world can support. But it is a concern that goes much further back to the eighteenth century when the cleric Thomas Malthus formulated his ideas on the subject.

Too Many People?

The English cleric Thomas Malthus published his ideas about what is often called the 'population explosion' in a book called *An Essay on the Principle of Population* in 1798. By then the Industrial Revolution in Europe had led to the movement of many thousands of people from rural communities to the growing cities, to escape the poverty of life in smaller agricultural villages and, hopefully, to gain employment in the burgeoning urban factories. These people were usually little better off as city-dwellers than they had been as farm labourers or smallholders. However, their supply of food was more dependable even if not of great quality, and with this greater security, the urban population grew.

This was also a time when the British Empire was built, as were the empires of several other European countries, and so the question of the population of subjects in the Continents of Asia, Africa and South

America arose. The imperial powers like Britain needed dependable numbers of people as workers – effectively slaves – to maintain the empire and to provide the goods on which Western prosperity depended. But the stability of the colonies depended on having enough, but not too many, subjects. Just as elsewhere, it was widely believed that the poor bred in an uncontrolled fashion. After all, no reliable forms of contraception were available.

Malthus believed that the problem would sort itself out. Population size will always be limited by the resources available, he suggested. So while it is true that doubling the size of a field may double the yield of crops or allow twice as many cattle to graze, human populations grow faster than this. If couples have four children instead of two, within two generations there are 16 mouths to feed, then 64, and so on. If some extra resources become available – maybe a larger field to cultivate – this may encourage an increase in family size. But they will nonetheless soon outstrip the resources available, for example in the amounts of food crops which they can grow. After an initial increase, the larger population in relation to food supply will inevitably mean that some people are going to starve. Malthus felt that after a period of time the population will stabilise at a new level which is similar, or only slightly higher, than the original level. This became known as the 'Malthusian trap' of economic development.

Not everyone agreed with Malthus about this rather fatalistic view of progress. Some critics argued that, as well as increasing demand for resources, an increase in population size would drive innovation and increase food and factory productivity, leading to economic growth. Probably there is some truth in both sides of the argument. But in reality, the importance of population growth has dominated economic thinking, at least in Western countries, ever since.

Today, overall global food production has kept pace with the growth of the world's population. But that does not mean that the food is distributed equally. About 811 million people don't have enough to eat even now, because food production and distribution isn't equitable. That is without taking into account the full force of the COVID-19 pandemic.

The WHO estimates that globally one in three people suffer from some form of malnutrition, and this includes not only those having inadequate food, an unbalanced diet lacking essential ingredients, but also those people who consume an excessive diet which is also unbalanced and unhealthy.

Even though an estimated 25,000 people die from hunger and related causes every day, there are other threats to survival that affect large numbers of people. Just 100 years ago, in affluent countries like the UK, many people who were reasonably healthy died of communicable diseases, infections caught from one another such as diphtheria, measles, tuberculosis, typhoid, cholera, smallpox, plague … . This list was very long. These diseases carried off many children and young adults, years before they were old enough to have developed chronic conditions such as cancer, heart disease or diabetes – the so-called non-communicable diseases (NCDs).

A century ago the treatments for infectious diseases were very limited. Usually doctors and other carers could do little for a patient except to keep them well-hydrated and cool, and hope that their immune system would catch up in time to win the battle over the invading bacteria or viruses.

In low- to middle-income countries, communicable diseases still take a terrible toll on lives. This may be because lack of adequate sanitation or clean water and crowded living conditions help infections to spread. As some infections are spread by insects, it may be because simple preventative measures such as mosquito nets are not available. Or it may be because treatments for infected individuals aren't available or are too expensive.

And while we still barely succeed in the battle against infections such as malaria or tuberculosis which have been known for a long time, new plagues of communicable disease arise from infectious agents, such as Ebola or Zika. So average life expectancy in low- to middle-income countries is much lower – for example in Sierra Leone today average life expectancy is 28 years less than it is in Singapore.

We were writing this book in the UK during the COVID-19 pandemic, when most European countries were in lockdown and we only left our homes to buy food or for other essential reasons. We were reminded that the simple act of washing our hands was vital.

Ignaz Semmelweis is thought to have been the first to notice the link between handwashing and infection in the mid-1800s in a maternity hospital setting, and we took a lot of convincing right up to the 1980s to make it part of everyday disease control. In 2020 we were encouraged to wash our hands for 20 seconds repeatedly, to wear a face mask and to keep at least 2 metres apart from others outside our immediate household. In a very short period of time, everyone became aware of some of the essential features of a pandemic – how the virus spread, the need to test those with symptoms of infection, to isolate them if they were COVID-positive and to track down the people with whom they had come into contact. Suddenly we all became experts on communicable disease.

If Malthus were here today, he might point to the higher infection rates, and so deaths, from COVID-19 in more densely populated places such as London, New York or Sao Paolo and say that this was exactly what his model predicted – allowing populations to increase excessively would almost certainly lead to a higher mortality in time. Higher COVID death rates are not due to lack of food, but they are associated with overcrowded living and poverty. These aspects of human life, and disease and death, are very unfairly distributed.

The majority of deaths around the world each year, almost three-quarters of deaths in fact, are caused by the so-called NCDs – far more than deaths from infectious diseases, accidents or conflict

---

There are some surprising aspects of this injustice, however, which are not widely appreciated.

The majority of deaths around the world each year, almost three-quarters of deaths in fact, are caused by the so-called NCDs – far more than deaths from infectious diseases, accidents or conflict. We might view this in a way as a success story for medicine and global health initiatives, as infectious diseases, accidents and violence have been the biggest killers in human populations for millennia. But once again the burden falls more heavily on low-resource populations. Eighty per cent of the deaths from NCDs occur each year in low- to middle-income countries.

The prevalent important NCDs are diseases of the heart and circulation, including heart attacks, strokes, high blood pressure and heart failure. This is followed by cancers and lung disease and by diabetes. NCDs develop slowly over the life course and by and large they can't be cured. There are many treatments that can reduce their impact, but usually once they have developed we have to live with them, although life expectancy is shorter. So today much attention among public health experts is being paid to how to prevent these NCDs developing in the first place.

The injustice in the risk of death from NCDs is seen not only around the globe, but even on a smaller scale. Life expectancy isn't the same everywhere in the UK, for example, and it even varies between places which are quite close.

There is a map of the London Underground, called *Lives on the Line*, which shows life expectancy for those people who live in the area around each tube station. The variations are dramatic. From Lancaster Gate to Mile End, a journey which takes 20 minutes on the Central Line, life expectancy falls by 12 years. By the same token, from Glasgow city centre, each stop on its local Argyle Line means a change in life expectancy of the local residents of about one year, at least for women. Why is this?

Greed, Gluttony and Sloth?

One reason is that the quality of medical care you can access depends on where you live. This might be because those living in wealthier parts of London or Glasgow can afford health insurance and access to better private medical care rather than rely on the UK's NHS. Or it might be because they have a higher level of education, and are more likely to find out about health risks, to take steps to prevent them, or to ask their primary healthcare physician or GP to screen them for common health conditions. Unfortunately, even the funding of NHS care varies between UK regions. The medical staff across these cities are equally qualified, experienced and dedicated but the support they receive, and the case-load they have to deal with, varies.

At the time of the founding in the UK of the NHS 70 years ago, social care services were also established, recognising that many elderly or other vulnerable people were not easily able to live at home or to look after themselves, especially if they were ill. There is much discussion about the funding of such care now, and it varies across regions too, with less access to affordable care available in deprived areas. At times of austerity it is highly susceptible to short-term government policies. But such regional differences are unlikely to account for variations in life expectancy across quite small distances, from local rail station to station.

Another potential answer lies in differences in lifestyle or behaviour. Those of us who smoke, get little physical exercise and have an unhealthy diet can expect to live shorter lives, because such factors have been clearly associated with risk of fatal diseases such as heart attacks, stroke, some forms of cancer and diabetes – the NCDs. Socio-economic conditions can be a powerful determinant of these aspects of lifestyle too, for example in terms of the financial resources needed to buy healthy food, employment or in leisure which gives time to take exercise.

Socio-economic status can vary over quite small distances like along a railway line. The importance of this factor is clear from the finding of the British Heart Foundation that the fall in deaths from cardiovascular disease, which has taken place year on year since the middle of the twentieth century, appears to have stopped. More people over 65 died of cardiovascular disease in 2017 than in 2014, bucking the trend which had been seen over previous five-year periods. This has been suggested to result from the longer-term effects of Britain's austerity policy, especially after the 2008 financial crisis, which has hit poorer members of society harder than more affluent people. And there are clear links between poverty, food insecurity and access to green spaces for exercise or relaxation.

Similar issues are seen in the USA where data show that average life expectancy has fallen in recent years, for the first time since records began.

So is adult lifestyle then the answer to why life expectancy differs across London or Glasgow, or indeed across the world, and why it has fallen in recent years? The simple answer is … that the answer is not that simple. There is no doubt that an unhealthy lifestyle shortens life by increasing the risk of cardiovascular disease, cancer and diabetes, to name three leading causes of death. And that death is more likely to occur if access to healthcare is limited and resources are scarce.

But this can't be the whole story.

> *In October 2020, Joan Hocquard, the oldest person in Britain at the time, died aged 112. Her nephew said she believed there was no secret to a long life and 'enjoyed butter and cream and she scoffed at the idea of dieting'*

We all know people who seem to lead blameless, healthy lives and yet are struck down by a fatal illness years before it would seem fair. Then again, there are older people who have smoked for years, take little physical exercise and have an unhealthy diet, and who live to a grand old age. In October 2020, Joan Hocquard, the oldest person in Britain at the time, died at the age of 112. Her nephew said that his aunt believed there was no secret to a long life and 'enjoyed butter and cream and she scoffed at the idea of dieting'. It seems as if some of us can lead an unhealthy lifestyle for years and get away with it.

This uncertainty is not helpful. If we don't know what causes a disease it isn't easy to prevent it. It has taken us all far too long to wake up to this problem. When the great and the good of the world got together to devise goals which together we should aim to achieve in the first 15 years of this new millennium, the so-called Millennium Development Goals, NCD prevention was not part of the plan.

In retrospect, this was a terrible omission. It was quickly appreciated in the first decade of the millennium, but by then it was too late to mount an international campaign to address the challenge, because countries had their sights set on achieving the Millennium Development Goals and dealing with the problems these posed.

It wasn't until the so-called Sustainable Development Goals were devised to follow on from the Millennium Development Goals from 2015 to 2030 that NCDs were clearly highlighted, by which time many opportunities had been missed and NCDs were reaching epidemic proportions in many countries.

The aim of one of the Sustainable Development Goals (Number 3) is to reduce the premature deaths from NCDs by a third by 2030. This is certainly ambitious, some might say over-ambitious. A recent review of progress made it clear that no country, whether low- to middle-income countries or higher-income countries, in the world is on course to meet this target – and that was before the COVID-19 pandemic, which changed the way funds were spent on health and had such dramatic economic consequences that we are now in a global economic recession.

But we still haven't answered the question of what is driving the epidemic of NCDs.

A Bridge Too Far

As you will have seen from this book, part of the answer to this question, perhaps the largest part, lies in our early development. It is those adaptive responses of the unborn baby that we discussed in Chapters 3 and 4, starting from the moment of conception.

Emphasising this was one of the reasons for writing this book. But we don't need to look at present patterns of disease to see how important early development is to later NCD risk. We get some very clear clues from history.

We already mentioned that, even today, large numbers of people die each day because of a lack of food. But the reality is even worse, because even if you don't die of starvation the effects of very poor nutrition can be life-altering for generations.

In the second half of 1944, pressure was increasing for an Allied invasion to liberate Northern Europe from its Nazi occupiers. Operation Market Garden was planned for September 1944, with the objective of capturing a series of bridges in the Netherlands which were vital to the occupying forces for the transport of troops and supplies. Starting with the dropping of large numbers of paratroopers, the battle raged from 17 to 25 September, but it ended in failure when the Allied forces were unable to cross the Rhine. The bridge at Arnhem was too heavily defended by German troops. It was a bridge too far, as in the title of the book by Cornelius Ryan and the feature film about this campaign.

Dutch resistance preparations and support for the Allied invasion had been strong, including the organisation of a strike by railway workers, designed to impede German communications and supplies. However, after the failure of Operation Market Garden the occupying forces carried out reprisals on the Dutch population, including a ban on food transport by rail to the western Netherlands.

At first it was possible to maintain supplies by transport on the canals, but unfortunately the winter of 1944–1945 was unusually cold and the canals froze. By November 1944, adult food rations were below 1,000 calories per day, compared to the recommended level of 2,500 calories per day for an adult woman. After the severe cold in January and February 1945 this ration had fallen to about 500 calories per day. This meant about 400 grams of bread and 1 kilogram of potatoes per week, with very small amounts of meat or cheese. Moreover, as there was virtually no gas or electricity, living conditions were bitterly cold.

The famine ended abruptly in May 1945 with the liberation of the Netherlands but its consequences were very long-lasting, even to the present day.

A crumb of comfort from this terrible story is that it has given rise to some deep insights into human development, which might not have been obtained otherwise. Like so much of health research, discoveries depend on having really reliable data. Despite the wartime privations and harsh conditions, doctors continued to keep detailed records of pregnancies and birth in the hospitals in the Netherlands.

Knowing the timing of the famine accurately has enabled researchers to examine the effects of a near-

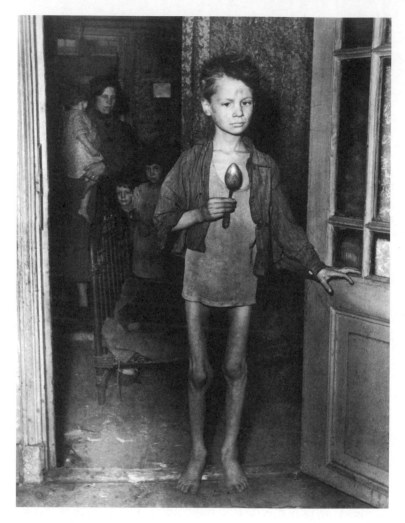

Figure 5.1 Henkie Holvast He was from the Tuinstraat and was severely undernourished during the 'Hunger Winter' in Amsterdam, the Netherlands (1944).
The Nederlands Fotomuseum, Inventory number MCM-100000, Image number 3d5a8745-c959-2954-89fd-5750712d183b.

starvation diet on women and their children, even down to the impact of the period in pregnancy when the undernutrition occurred. Overall, the babies born to women exposed to the famine were smaller than those before or after it, but only by about 200 grams if their mothers were starved in later pregnancy. Starvation in early or mid-pregnancy had no, or only a very small, effect. Clearly the fetus was able to sustain its growth, albeit at the expense of the mother's nutrition, in the face of this extreme challenge.

Because the Dutch doctors kept detailed records of these births throughout the period, despite the harsh conditions imposed by the Nazi occupiers, it has been possible to follow up the children of the Dutch Hunger Winter to investigate longer-term effects on their health throughout their lives.

Children famished in early gestation went on as adults to have a substantially higher risk of many NCDs

---

The results are dramatic. Even though they appeared to have coped with the challenge of poor nutrition in the womb, those children famished in early gestation went on as adults to have a substantially higher risk of many NCDs, including high blood pressure, diabetes and some mental ill-health conditions. They were affected more severely in this way than those individuals who were famished in later gestation. The research fitted with the growing realisation that many of the body's structures and physiological functions are set up in early gestation.

The principle established by the Dutch Hunger Winter of early adaptive responses by the developing embryo or fetus having possible later consequences has been confirmed several times in other parts of the world.

In China, in the Great Leap Forward from 1958 to 1962, in which Mao Zedong's Chinese Communist Party attempted to generate communes for the population at the expense of more traditional agriculture, between 18 and 45 million people are thought to have died. The children and grandchildren of those who were starved but survived are now experiencing an epidemic of obesity, diabetes and other NCDs.

Something similar is emerging in West Africa in the descendants of those caught up in the Nigerian civil war of 1967–1970 in which as many as two million Biafran people died. There seems to be a pattern here, of NCD risk being passed across generations. If it isn't due to fixed genetic inheritance, what is the basis of this passage?

The Musical Score Is Not the Performance

Even if you are a very gifted musician, you can't tell just by looking at the score of a piece, for example the notes for a singer or for playing by other instruments, what it will sound like when performed. It may be faster or more melancholy that you anticipated. The singer may not quite hit a high note, or one of the instruments may be too loud and make her hard to hear. Every time the piece is played it will sound slightly different, even though the notes for the parts written down in the score are the same. A band may play the same song over and over in a recording studio until they get a version they like, and even then it is often edited and manipulated electronically.

In some ways how our bodies develop shares similarities with a musical performance. As we said earlier in the book, the genes we each inherited from our parents are fixed in our developing cells, and we could think of them as rather like the musical score. But how those genes work varies according to which cell of the body they are in, and from one moment to the next. These sorts of things affect

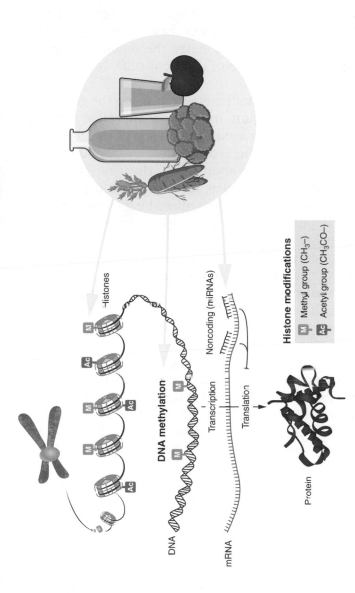

Figure 5.2 Epigenetics and nutrition Nutrition is one factor that can direct tiny modifications of our DNA from the earliest stages of our development. These 'epigenetic' modifications don't alter the unique genetic makeup each of us inherited but change the way it operates in making the proteins that build our bodies and make them work.

how the genes are switched on or off and so the proteins that are made by the cells. There is nothing very surprising about this – after all, there have to be mechanisms which allow the same set of genes, the genome, to be used to generate a wide range of different cells, from brain to bladder to blood.

The switching mechanisms which act on the genome to control gene 'expression' in this way are called epigenetic processes, meaning around or on top of the genes. The word was coined by the Scottish developmental biologist Conrad Waddington in about 1942. His idea wasn't fashionable at the time and was rather overlooked for many years, even though it was recognised by scientists interested in development that something like epigenetic processes must be operating.

The revolution in thinking came about in the late twentieth century when it became possible to measure the chemical processes which are involved in epigenetic switching. It turned out that these are quite simple, but they are very widespread – operating at millions of points in the genome. Even more exciting was the discovery that epigenetic processes can be altered by factors such as nutrition, oxygen levels, hormones, drugs, toxins and so on, leaving epigenetic 'marks' on the genome which can have long-lasting effects on how genes work. And it turned out that such marks can be measured in white blood cells, in a swab of cells from the mouth, in hair and nails – all tissues which are accessible.

In Chapter 3 we saw that the development of some organs occurs during development at specific times. For example, the number of cells in our hearts and the number of filtering units in our kidneys are established before we are born and can't be changed later. The so-called plasticity of development operates over critical periods of time, and it is time-limited. This is when the epigenetic marks are being made on top of the genetic code.

The consequences of these new – or re-invented, if we give Waddington the credit he deserves – discoveries are that measuring epigenetic marks, in for example blood cells, can reveal information about a person's early life, even during their first 1,000 days. And that information can tell us about such things as their heart and kidney development. And then, because the development of those organs relates to their later risk of NCDs, epigenetic marks can be linked to later risk of ill health.

Research into epigenetics is now very active and widespread. But to return to the story of the Dutch Hunger Winter, it has shown the mechanisms by which famine during particular periods of the first 1,000 days can be associated with later risk of ill health. It has even been possible to show that some epigenetic processes appear to be passed across to the next generation too, affecting the grandchildren of those pregnant women starved during the Second World War.

And more recent studies have shown that epigenetic marks measured at birth even in healthy normal babies today can be linked to their mother's diet and weight, and in turn to how their cardiovascular systems and the amount of fat in their bodies develop through childhood.

Waddington would be amazed at the extent to which his word epigenetics has changed our ideas about our early development.

I Didn't See *That* Coming

We started this chapter by emphasising that the world changes around us, and by us, over time. It seems a tall order to expect the adaptive responses that the fetus in the womb makes to the mother's environment to be relevant for life. So some developmental changes that it has made may well turn out to be poorly suited to the world in which it lives now. Shit happens.

The long-term intergenerational impact of the Dutch Hunger Winter did not become clear until many years after the Second World War. Food was scarce at times in many parts of wartime Europe and so you can see how well-meaning efforts to prioritise the needs of the pregnant woman and the growing fetus in the post-war years would have reinforced the myth that the pregnant woman needed to 'eat for two'. This is still sometimes said today.

We now know that this is definitely unhealthy. True, not enough food or an unbalanced diet will affect growth of the baby, but 'eating for two' won't make the fetus grow better. It will only make the mother gain too much weight, which isn't healthy either for her or her baby. If the baby is also bigger at birth, this will be because it has too much body fat. The woman who is obese, or the woman with a type of diabetes which occurs in pregnancy (gestational diabetes) is also more likely to give birth to an overweight baby, which may not only be hard to deliver but has risks of later ill health too.

Generally speaking, all our bodies get less good at controlling themselves as we get older. With age, we all get a little less adaptable to the world we live in and less resilient to the things that can challenge our health, such as poor diet, sedentary lifestyle or stress. This increases the risk of NCDs in particular, and it is perhaps no surprise that most of us will die from one form of NCD or another. But how soon we succumb to these NCDs, the trajectory of risk, differs between people.

The fetus who is undernourished and growing a little less well – but not dramatically growth-restricted – is not preparing as well to meet the challenge of the rich and unbalanced diet that is now so common

We've already said in Chapter 1 that genes from your parents and your lifestyle don't explain it all. We now know that how you are put together during early development, which is different for each organ system, sets up your trajectory, the rate of increase, of NCD risk as you get older. The fetus who is undernourished and growing a little less well – and we emphasise that they are not dramatically growth-restricted – is not preparing as well to meet the challenge of the rich and unbalanced diet that is now so common. So then, as a child the way their body works will be 'mismatched', less able to respond to the junk diet they are eating. They are biologically less in control and their health is more at risk.

This way of thinking represents a seismic change in how we view our control over our bodies in the world in which we find ourselves.

Man Hands on Misery to Man

So, if early development is so important in later risk of NCDs, then are the places in the world where early development is poorest also those places where the majority of NCDs occur? The answer is 'Yes'. We said above that it was true of countries such as China or Nigeria where the population was exposed to armed conflict and severe undernutrition in the last century.

We see exactly the same situation in many low- to middle-income countries. There are many factors affecting early development: poor nutrition; limited access to healthcare, especially for women and children; poor sanitation; teenage pregnancies and short intervals between pregnancies; environmental degradation; low levels of vaccination … the list goes on.

So we can see how babies born today in many low- to middle-income countries are likely to be potentially mismatched – influenced by something from this list of factors which affects their development and then makes them less able to cope with challenges to their health later. The tragedy is that even a small degree of economic progress, which should theoretically make the lives of a population better in the long run, can risk making the mismatch greater, and the NCD risk worse, for some of its members in the shorter term.

Take sanitation for example. Unclean water, possibly polluted with sewage, is a major of cause of gastro-enteritis in many settings, and in children the resulting dehydration, malnutrition and long-term inflammation of the intestines can be fatal. Places where the water is polluted are often inaccessible and perhaps not economically very productive, so there is little incentive to improve the situation. Let's say, however, that a philanthropic organisation generates the funds to provide water purification, and pipes to supply clean water and to dispose of sewage effectively. There will be better health, economic progress and things will look better. It may be worth providing a better access route for trade, in terms of sale of produce from the region and of goods from outside.

This is all great, except that along with such progress come other things. Magazines, television and the internet promote an ideal life which is often based on a Western, high-income country model. And this includes fast food and sedentary pursuits. The first small retail outlets in such a region won't be selling fresh fruit, fish and high fibre cereals or eggs and milk. These foods are hard to transport and have a short shelf-life. They'll be selling fast foods, high in fat and salt, and highly sweetened drinks. These are easily preserved and transported and need no preparation to consume, and they are usually fairly cheap and tasty. But they are not very healthy. The children and adults in this region of the low- to middle-income country

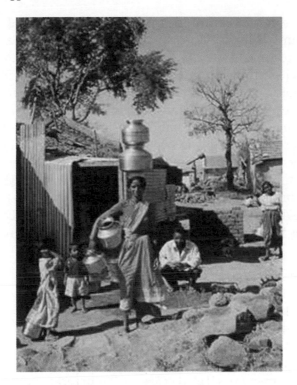

Figure 5.3 Young woman and her family in rural India
Courtesy of Professors Caroline Fall and Chittaranjan Yajnik and the Pune Maternal Nutrition Study.

whose early development was poorest will be mismatched to the health challenge posed by such food and so at greater risk of obesity and NCDs.

Then, as if this problem were not enough, it gets worse.

Despite NCDs being called 'non'-communicable, they are the opposite. Their risk is communicated across generations

As we noted before, despite NCDs being called 'non'-communicable, they are in fact just the opposite. Their risk is communicated, at least across generations. And as we discussed earlier, this is not predominantly via inheriting genetic defects. The diabetes now so common in many countries, and the special form of diabetes occurring in pregnancy (gestational diabetes), can increase the risk of diabetes in the offspring by almost tenfold. So children of mothers with diabetes are much more likely to have diabetes themselves as young adults, and to pass that risk on to their children in turn.

It really does look like the idea behind Philip Larkin's famous poem about parents called 'This Be The Verse':

> They fuck you up, your mum and dad.
> They may not mean to, but they do.
> ... ...
> Man hands on misery to man.
> It deepens like a coastal shelf.
> Get out as early as you can,
> And don't have any kids yourself.
>
> (Extract from *High Windows* by Philip Larkin published by
> Faber and Faber Ltd. Reproduced with permission.)

Get out as early as you can? Opportunities for changing or even leaving poor living conditions are limited for many of the world's 1.2 billion adolescents. And we wouldn't want to deny them the opportunity to have a family of their own.

In addition, although in higher-income countries populations are getting older on average, in many low- to middle-income countries the opposite is true. In sub-Saharan Africa the percentage of the population who are adolescents is rising – it's almost 25% in some places – partly because infectious diseases such as HIV/AIDS have claimed the lives of many of their parents. Supporting these adolescents, to help them not to develop NCDs, and not to pass on a greater risk of NCDs in turn to their children, is an enormous challenge.

But it is a challenge which we all must face. In terms of global health, humanitarian and economic consequences, turning our backs on this challenge is not an option we can contemplate.

As we saw in Chapter 2, pregnancy and childbirth are still very dangerous times in the lives of women in low- to middle-income countries. Great strides have been made in reducing the death toll from this natural event – which should be a source of joy rather than fear – but far too many women still die around the birth of their child.

In low- to middle-income countries the commonest cause of maternal death after delivering the baby is haemorrhage. Such bleeding can be stopped if staff are trained to act quickly – and so the condition only accounts for a few maternal deaths in higher-income countries. As we said in Chapter 2, many of these deaths are associated with health problems which affect women before they became pregnant, such as diabetes, anaemia or cardiovascular disease. These conditions could, and should, have been treated before. Then lives would have been saved. And these disasters illustrate our point about the transmission of NCD risk and its threatening consequences across generations very well.

But those of us who live in higher-income countries shouldn't be complacent. In the UK the number of children living in poverty has increased every year over the last 10 years. They are now over four million – about one in three children. This number could easily rise to 50% by the middle of this century if current trends continue, and the situation has been made worse by the COVID-19 pandemic and the financial recession which resulted.

Even before the pandemic, in 2019, 70% of these children were in working families. They clearly have low income, and many of them live in deprived urban areas and especially among ethnic minorities. But they are not the children of parents who are unemployed and struggling to live on the UK government's much-criticised system of benefits.

> *Children in lower socio-economic families have a greater risk of being obese by the time they start primary school, and even more so by the time they move to secondary school.*

The problem extends beyond that. Children in lower socio-economic families have a greater risk of being obese by the time they start primary school, and even more so by the time they move to secondary school; and so a greater risk of chronic illnesses such as the NCDs, later. Needless to say, their diets and lifestyles are not healthy.

The life course trajectory of disease risks which children living in poverty in higher-income countries have been forced to follow is very similar to that of many children in low- to middle-income countries. We can see the evidence for this from the statistics which show that child mortality in the first year of life in the UK is rising again, after having fallen continuously for the last 100 years.

Women and Children Last

NCDs are major killers with enormous – and growing – economic, humanitarian and social implications. To prevent NCDs, their risk factors need to be reduced. Why then is so little being done to prevent them? Why is no country on track to meet the target internationally agreed in 2015?

We hope, from what we have said in this book, that it is evident that the NCD prevention agenda starts long before the moment of conception, and involves both parents. NCD risks are passed across generations, because babies and children inherit a biology which is more than just determined by their inherited genes and which leads to a more or less risky health profile into old age.

This raises a very important ethical concern, because these young members of the next generation, and those as yet unborn or not even conceived, have no choice or control over the factors which set the beginnings of such risk. We have a duty to protect them.

Not only that, but it is a sad truth that women and children are the sections of the population most often at the bottom of the food chain when it comes to resources for health, education and social justice. They may have little agency, the ability to act to change things, almost as if they are non-citizens. This is of course exactly what women were in the days before they were given the vote.

'Women and children first!' might be the command to preserve life when passengers struggle to get into the lifeboats of a sinking ship, but it's definitely 'women and children last' in many other situations. This is sadly true in every society, to a greater or lesser degree.

The triumphs of second wave feminism in helping many women to decide if, when and with whom to conceive a child have not been translated universally into every society. And the agenda of third wave feminism barely features in many places, so women are as powerless as they were 100 years ago. They suffer much of the same discrimination and the consequences of inequality in opportunities, education, pay, control over their reproductive lives – and health.

Women make many contributions to the economies of the world through unpaid labour – child rearing, care of elderly relatives and household chores for example. Even the paid jobs which women undertake, often in the more informal economies of countries, frequently do not provide paid sick leave, maternity leave or support for breastfeeding.

These inequalities are amplified in times of socioeconomic shock like the 2008 global financial crisis and the current COVID-19 pandemic. During the pandemic women have been found to be more likely to contract the infection than men, even though they are less likely to die from it. Why is this? Probably because they are more likely to be carrying out menial jobs which involve cleaning and disinfecting, going to market, and caring for children and older relatives who can't necessarily be expected to keep high standards of personal hygiene.

In the UK, the value of unpaid household service work, largely carried out by women, contributes as much as the whole non-financial corporate sector, equivalent to over 60% of GDP

Such work is often unremunerated, which means that it does not contribute to measures of economic production such as the Gross Domestic Product (GDP). Governments care about GDP because the earnings it represents will also relate to taxation and because profit leads to investment and so further growth in GDP. However, in the UK, the value of unpaid household service work, largely carried out by women, contributes as much as the whole non-financial corporate sector, equivalent to over 60% of GDP. Much more truthful measures of real value to society are those such as the Socio-demographic Index which includes factors like the number of years of schooling and fertility of females.

The COVID-19 pandemic has worsened economic prospects across the world on a massive scale. Globally, 42–66 million people are now in extreme poverty with women, children and adolescents more affected due to the lack of social, financial and health protection. It's estimated that there has been a 37% increase in maternal deaths and a 28% increase in stillbirths. Many girls have stopped attending school and there are reports of an increase in child marriages in some societies. Fertility rates have risen, with access to contraception reduced and in over a hundred low- to middle-income countries it is calculated that there have been nearly 1.4 million more unintended pregnancies. Domestic violence to women has increased by 30% to up to 300% depending on the country.

Over 17 million children have missed their scheduled diphtheria, pertussis and tetanus vaccinations and 94 million children their measles vaccine. So the impact on infectious disease rates will soon be felt. An additional 67 million children became severely malnourished or wasted in 2020, compared to 2019 figures and, as we explained above, they will grow up to be a potentially mismatched generation, with increased risk of NCDs too.

When societies are most challenged by a threat, as with the COVID-19 pandemic, it is women who increasingly have to clean up the mess, and whose lives suffer from setbacks in societal progress made before. Their jobs are often the first to be lost when times are tough, and return more slowly than men's when economic recovery starts.

Young women are literally at the bottom of the food chain too, often having the poorest and most insecure nutrition of the family, while sometimes having to be engaged in heavy physical work in agriculture until late pregnancy.

One of the most important factors in addressing this issue is education, because teenage girls who are allowed to remain in school are more likely to be empowered, less likely to become pregnant at an early age and more likely to gain paid employment. The latter, as opposed to unpaid or very poorly paid work similar to zero-hours contracts, can help to support them and their families in having a healthier lifestyle, and makes them more independent and visible as drivers of the future economy.

Motherhood is the anvil on which all gender inequalities are forged

---

Rachel Cusk, *A Life's Work*

The novelist Rachel Cusk wrote one of the best memoirs of motherhood, called *A Life's Work*. In it she says: 'Motherhood is the anvil on which all gender inequalities are forged'. Many women, in many parts of the world, would agree with this.

Just about every society disadvantages women, in terms of their careers, their freedom and even their fundamental rights when they become mothers. Mothers are held responsible for many aspects of the lives of their children, their partners and sometimes other members of the family too. This is the kind of retrospective, backward-looking 'blame and shame' responsibility that is so unhelpful.

What is needed is a forward-looking, prospective idea of responsibility that recognises that women are biologically equipped to be mothers and that society values this and will support them without their paying penalties in other areas of their lives.

We have uncovered probably the most important reason why progress towards reducing the burden of NCDs worldwide has been so slow. Because the trajectory of risk for NCDs starts during our first 1,000 days, reducing the risk requires nothing less than recognition that women and their partners must be helped to do so. Women need the basic freedom, the knowledge and the resources – in other words the agency – to exercise such responsibility. We tackle these issues in the next chapter.

Unfortunately, the evidence for this life course trajectory of risk of NCDs, starting in very early development, and of the transmission of risk across the generations, has taken a very long time to be recognised. In fact, in many quarters – from the media to Departments of Health and doctors' offices – it still has not been recognised. So what are we to do?

6 THE GIFT

Who's in Charge Here?

So it would seem that we need to end our story with a call to action. But who is it aimed at?

Supporting and empowering women and their partners during the preconception and pregnancy periods of their lives, and the early years of their children's lives, sounds like something which should be high on the list of priorities for government health policy-makers, doesn't it?

Shouldn't an issue which affects everyone in a population be the easiest type of challenge for a government to address? Every citizen over the age of two and alive today has gone through 1,000 days of development. And very many citizens are, or will be, parents. So we might think that making the first 1,000 days the best it can be for everyone would be just about the easiest policy to carry out, and probably the most popular.

But it's not like that. We need to examine why. Even when the facts are very clear and acknowledged, government policy does not necessarily change. Policy-making is inevitably about choices between options – for example, in the UK, in the temporary recovery from the COVID-19 pandemic in England in the summer of 2020, policy initially prioritised the opening of pubs and restaurants to restart the economy over supporting children's education and wellbeing by opening schools.

There are always factions within and outside government who support a particular strategy, and these can compete and be equally vociferous. They may have influential champions and may gain considerable public support, making them hard to ignore. As a result, strategies can sometimes develop as a result of a dramatic and well-publicised event, at the expense of a long established, carefully researched agenda.

In addition, policy-makers do not respond well to problems which do not have a clear solution. They usually ask experts in a particular field for their opinions on a solution, but very often these experts don't agree on what this might be. So, the issue gets parked for the time being.

As a result, policy-makers can seem slow or unwilling to act. They know that they can't do much about our inherited genes, unless they embark on some massive eugenics programme to breed out supposedly 'bad' genes from the population, which would be tantamount to the pre-war fascist agenda to breed a 'master race'. And we really hope that this is not an option in today's world.

Another reason for policy inaction is that the developmental story we have told in this book reads like a novel which describes the lives of a family across generations. It's an epic like Leo Tolstoy's *War and Peace*, with interwoven life stories over a long timeline. Governments don't like long stories: they are elected to govern for a few years and have to show successful outcomes in that time.

Then we have to consider the options open to a government for addressing *any* challenge. Legislation is one, but promoting the idea of the 'best first 1,000 days' does not lend itself to legislation as easily as other things which are good for us. We can support laws which state that everyone must wear a seatbelt in a car, a mask in a shop during a pandemic or that smoking isn't permitted in enclosed public places. But governments shy away from interfering with more personal aspects of our lives – and it is possible to view the conception and development of the next generation as a very personal matter.

> *In reality, health challenges which affect a smaller number of individuals can often be easier to address than those which affect public health more widely*

In reality, health challenges which affect a smaller number of individuals can often be easier to address than those which affect public health more widely. For example, if a drug taken by pregnant women is found to produce adverse effects on the fetus, as happened with thalidomide in the UK, recommendations can quickly be made to prohibit its use and the individuals affected can be given help and compensation, however inadequate that may seem. This will require resource, but it's relatively straightforward because the individuals affected are known and any intervention is likely to be widely supported and popular. The same is often not the case for public health measures which affect a population more widely.

Governments shy away from appearing like a 'nanny state', telling their electorate how to behave because they know what is best for them. Neo-liberal politicians don't like such control, any more than they do regulating financial markets. And governments find it hard to moderate swells in populist, even alt-right, movements with strongly held extreme views.

So without clear policies in place for promoting health in the first 1,000 days, where does that leave us?

Homer Simpson's Advice

The challenge of making our first 1,000 days healthy goes beyond saying that it is difficult. It's not just that it's hard to address this challenge in a country, whether a low- to middle-income country or a high-income country: it's more that there's little motivation to do so.

Rather like Homer in *The Simpsons* cartoon who remarks: 'If something's hard to do, it's not worth doing'.

Without motivation not much will happen, and any new initiatives won't be popular.

We've already set out why we think this is not popular with government and policy-makers. But who else is it not popular with? Unfortunately, the answer to this question is: 'just about everybody'.

It's unpopular with young people, mothers and parents and especially many young women. They are tired of being told that being overweight must be dealt with. They are fed up with feeling blamed for yet another aspect of their behaviour, or even their biology, over which they actually have very little control. And after all, women have been going through pregnancy and looking after young children for hundreds of thousands of years without this fundamental aspect of their lives being judged, found wanting and made the focus for annoying, even if well-meaning, interventions.

Try Googling 'What should I eat in pregnancy?' Which of the million or so links which pop up is the right one to follow?

And it's not as if there's clear agreement among the doctors, public health officials and scientists on what young women should actually be doing in any case. Try Googling 'What should I eat in pregnancy?' Which of the million or so links which pop up is the right one to follow?

Maybe it's best to ask the doctor or the midwife. But this question isn't popular with doctors or midwives either. They of course may have Googled the issue too and they may have accessed some of the publications in medical and scientific journals. In the UK they should also have read the guidance from organisations such as Public Health England (now the National Institute for Health Protection) or the NHS, and in other countries, from their own public health institutions. But it's a complex issue and there seems to be no simple answer. There are other more pressing issues which motivate them more.

Of course, healthcare professionals can advise a young woman who is planning to become pregnant, or who has recently found that she is pregnant, to eat a healthy diet, not to smoke, keep active and consume alcohol in small amounts if at all. But every one of these recommendations raises questions about why and how. Why is the woman's diet not healthy, for example? Perhaps it's because she doesn't know what a healthy diet is; or because she feels she can't afford it; or perhaps her partner won't eat it; or maybe it's just too difficult to prepare bearing in mind all the other challenges she's facing in her life right now. How can she change this?

This is a vast far-reaching question which the doctor almost certainly does not have either the time, the training or the resources to address. Medical students in many countries, including the UK, receive little if any specific training in nutrition. It's not a clinical specialty, like, say, obstetrics and gynaecology, or paediatrics.

Obesity is now so common in the population that it is quite likely that the doctor, or midwife or nurse, is overweight or obese themselves. If they don't feel that they appear to be a good role model, it can be difficult to tackle this issue with their patient. Obesity is so stigmatised, so much a matter of blame and placing the responsibility on us all as individuals for making bad personal choices about our lifestyles, that it becomes a taboo subject.

You might say that we should have written a guide for doctors and other healthcare professionals, to help them to focus on their roles in supporting development, based on the new knowledge about development in our first 1,000 days which has emerged over recent decades. Maybe some of them would read it and think how they might change their clinical practice.

But we haven't written that book. There are plenty of academic articles and even textbooks which provide that information. We know because we and our colleagues contributed to some of them. No, we understood that this book needed a different purpose, addressing the urgent need to call out the message about the importance of early development to a much wider audience.

If healthcare professionals aren't equipped, and politicians are disinclined, to act, the onus is back on the individual woman and her partner. Even if they understand the need to act, for example to prevent future risk of NCDs in themselves and even more so in their children, and even if they can overcome a sense that they are somehow to blame, what are they to do?

The Known and the Unknown

Based on a large amount of recent scientific research, we know that there are factors of which many of us aren't aware which have a profound influence on our health for life. They are passed on from our parents and start to take effect from the moment that each of us was conceived.

The first few chemical reactions, the epigenetic and physical processes in the fertilised egg mark the start of the life of every person and are the early steps on the pathway to being healthy which each of us follows.

As we've seen, these processes at conception are far more than just the selection of genes which we have inherited from our parents. It's too simplistic to say that how we'll develop and how we'll turn out is a genetic lottery, a lucky 'pick' from a list of possibilities.

Our development over our first 1,000 days involves a myriad of highly controlled processes, responding to inputs and cues from our surroundings, and triggering unconscious decisions about how to shape our development

---

Rather, the function of the different set of genes which each of us has inherited from our parents at conception is influenced by the environment and lives of our parents. This influence is particularly strong during our first 1,000 days and involves a myriad of highly controlled processes, responding to inputs and cues from our surroundings, and triggering unconscious decisions about how to shape our development.

The discoveries we have described in this book about how our early development influences our risk of NCDs later in our lives are important – if only because, statistically, it is the NCDs which are most likely to prove fatal for the majority of us, all around the world. In addition, as the current COVID-19 pandemic has shown, having an NCD such as high blood pressure or diabetes increases the risk of hospitalisation and death if we are unlucky enough to contract the infection. So communicable and non-communicable diseases cannot really be considered separately.

The more we think about this, the more we realise that right now we are less in control of our health than we thought.

This isn't to say that our actions and behaviour don't affect our health and our life chances: if we smoke, abuse alcohol or drugs, have an unbalanced diet, become obese and take little physical exercise we risk our health and may reduce our life expectancy. But even then, we know that as individuals we respond to these health threats in different ways. And as researchers have discovered in recent decades, these different ways of responding are partly set up in our first 1,000 days of development. We carry the epigenetic memory of our early development with us as we respond to these later health threats.

We're obsessed with the idea of being in complete control of our bodies and what happens to them, when in reality we know that this isn't possible

This line of argument can seem frightening. We don't like to admit that crucial aspects of our health aren't under our control. But maybe that's because we're obsessed with the idea of being in complete control of our bodies and what happens to them, when in reality we know that this isn't possible. We know that the underlying physiological processes which operate in our bodies aren't under our command. We can't control how we digest our lunch, how fast our heart beats or the level of our blood pressure. This might not matter most of the time because, despite our differences, our bodies usually 'tick over' quite nicely and regulate their function very well.

Even if we can't control this autonomy of our bodies, we can influence our body processes. We know that if we leave it until the last minute before dashing to an important meeting, we are likely to arrive breathless and feeling as if our heart is jumping in our chest. Or if we consume a large meal just before going to bed that we are likely to be kept awake by indigestion. We can do things like allowing more time to get to meetings for less stress, altering our mealtimes, even changing what we eat and the exercise we take.

But the amount of benefit we get from these changes differs between us, in terms of how well we control our response to stress, how changes in diet or exercise change our body shape or ability to control blood pressure or blood glucose.

These differences between us in how we can influence our body processes tend to get more noticeable the older we get. But of course, as we've seen in this book, how these differences are set up in the first place is very important.

In the setting of many of our body structures and control processes in early life we owe everything to our parents. Whether they knew it or not, they passed on vital information about the world they inhabited, and about their behaviour and health in that world. With the best of unconscious intentions, the signals they transmitted to us helped each of us to develop in what would most likely be the best way.

This is especially true of the challenges which we humans have faced many times in our evolutionary past, such as famine. Young children are better equipped physiologically to survive famine if they were on the small side at birth. A signal about the need to be prepared to face famine seems to have been passed to them before birth, changing their body's metabolic processes to run lean and mean. In a study of Jamaican children, a lighter birthweight by around 300 grams, possibly due to poor nourishment in the womb, and a 'metabolism' that had developed to operate in a meagre environment, made them better able to cope with periods of malnutrition as children. It is possible that something of the same sort occurs if the mother is exposed to a higher level of stress during pregnancy.

We're all potentially mismatched to our environment

But we are starting to appreciate that our development can't equip us so well to deal with the relatively newer – in evolutionary terms – aspects of our present environment which we face. We're all potentially mismatched to our environment now. As we saw in Chapter 5, shit happens.

We need some inside information, a warning signal so that we can develop in a way that will help us to face the challenges of a brave new world which we'll inhabit after birth.

Obesity and unhealthy behaviours, poor diet or exposure to toxic chemicals in the environment can send signals between generations which do not promote healthy development. Perhaps these challenges, as with conditions such as gestational diabetes which were rare until recently, are so novel in evolutionary terms that they take our development by surprise. And our parents, who

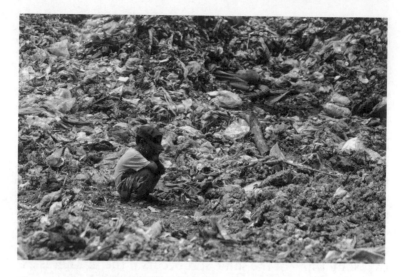

Figure 6.1 Environmental toxins and our children Toxins and
pollution depicted in this landfill site in Alue Liem in Lhokseumawe,
Indonesia (2021) are clearly unhealthy. Less well appreciated is that
the effects of toxic chemicals in the environment can send signals
between generations, perpetuating unhealthy development.
Azwar Ipank/AFP/Getty Images.

consciously and biologically want the best for their children, are not able to send appropriate warning signals in
the first 1,000 days.

The important point is that, whatever the signals our
parents sent us during those 1,000 days, we need to think
about that time in our lives and how it may have altered
the path to health or disease we now follow.

We need to know about this, each of us, if we want to
be in control.

The Personal Is Political

The strapline of the (as some people feel) slightly inferior
second *Jaws* movie was 'This time it's personal'.

But as will be apparent from what we've said throughout this book, we prefer the feminist slogan 'The personal

is political' to emphasise that as individuals we only have as much agency – our ability to act to change things – as the society in which we live and its over-arching political ideology will allow.

This does not mean that the only chance we have to change political thinking for the better is when we elect our political leaders. Society is much more than that and has needs and values that don't just surface at election time. There is a bigger, loosely defined force called public opinion and it grows daily through social media even if this does not always lead to a consensus among the members of a society. Depending on where you live and other circumstances, public opinion could change policy in the UK or in other countries.

During the COVID-19 pandemic the UK government was keen to be seen to be 'following the science', which was an outward demonstration to the voting public of valuing scientific fact. But policy-making struggled to keep up with the rapidly emerging scientific data and to balance it against the needs and desires of the public that were being voiced and some deeply entrenched political ideology. Communication broke down at times, and journalists queried whether the UK government was in touch with the opinions of its electorate. Across the world there was a range of responses by national governments, from authoritarian impositions of control over movement and behaviour, to more liberal delegation of responsibility to individuals, and even denial that the problem existed.

This raises the question of how much the 'general public' value or understand contemporary science. In 2019, just before the COVID pandemic, the UK government sponsored a survey of public attitudes to science. About half of those interviewed felt that science was important to society, and they felt well informed about science. This was an improvement on a previous government survey in 2014. But, compared with 2014, in 2019 there was a downward trend in the extent to which people in the UK felt that science is relevant to their daily lives. The picture is a little better for younger members of the population, who may be the parents of tomorrow. As authors of this book, we were not surprised by these figures – they fit with work we have been doing at the University of Southampton for several years.

Youth Voice

Development over our first 1,000 days is an amazing time in our lives, not least because it's a period which none of us remembers. It's a time of great potential, because during this stage every human being will develop to be a unique person. It is also a time of risks. And those risks continue, sometimes in the form of unhealthy behaviour, right through life. Sometimes, though, they peak during adolescence.

There are a few really important things to say about adolescence.

Adolescence goes on much longer than we thought. The WHO describes it as ending at age 19, but some paediatricians in the UK believe that it should be at 24. Scientists studying the brain have shown that our brains are not fully mature until our mid-twenties, at least in terms of our ability to make responsible decisions. Is this a surprise? Some might say that we must have known this for ages – after all, we call the last of our teeth to appear, usually in our mid-twenties, wisdom teeth.

To say that adolescence is the transition from childhood to adult life is to oversimplify it enormously. Adolescence is a time of dramatic changes in life. It's a time of alterations in our bodies, including a rapid growth in height and sexual maturation. And it can be a time of immense emotional upheaval too – in part because of the effects on our brains of the hormonal changes which are going on in our bodies.

In the middle of the nineteenth century adolescence wasn't recognised. The school leaving age was 10 in England and very few teenagers had any formal education after that. Most had to work, sometimes to support relatives or younger siblings. Many teenagers were soon parents themselves. They had to be more responsible, for themselves and the consequences of their behaviour, than most teenagers need to be today. Even so, globally even today 44 of every 1,000 births are to girls aged 15–19 years old.

In most developed countries, adolescence is a time when new opportunities open up, but it can also be incredibly frustrating too.

Teenagers are starting to feel autonomous, responsible and pretty much grown up, and yet there are so many things they aren't permitted to do: in most societies you can't vote, drive a car or drink in a bar until the age of 18. These restrictions may have been placed to protect adolescents at the time in their lives when they move from the innocence of childhood to the experience of adulthood through a phase of risk-taking, rebellious behaviour or even downright courting of danger. The commonest causes of death among adolescent males in most countries are accidents and physical violence. And adolescence is also a time when the risk of suicide increases frighteningly.

But while risk-taking is just the kind of behaviour which keeps older members of society awake at night, adolescents sometimes can't see the restrictions imposed on them in any positive light. An enlightened parent might realise that the mood swings and apparently antisocial behaviour of their teenage son or daughter is not completely under conscious control.

In our work we look at this 'risky' time in life in another way.

Encouraging young people to think outside the box, to think about what makes them healthy into older age, is one of the aims of the 'LifeLab' initiative in Southampton,

UK. In a collaboration between Southampton University's Institute of Developmental Sciences, the General Hospital and the city's schools, we set up a dedicated classroom and laboratory in the main hospital building. Over recent years more than 11,500 13–15-year-old school students have come to LifeLab to engage in hands-on experiments and to find out about the science behind health messages.

LifeLab would never work if it did not support the teachers in the schools involved and if it did not provide activities which can be linked to the school curriculum. But it provides a stimulating and thought-provoking experience rather than straightforward didactic teaching. Its strapline is '*Me, my health and my children's health*'. Our research shows that even a year after their visit, the students have retained many of the ideas about the importance of healthy behaviours at this time in their lives, and they have a more critical attitude to their own behaviour. Perhaps even more important, the programme creates young champions to spread these ideas to their peers.

These results have made us redouble our efforts, with colleagues, to open our Research Institute doors to young people. For several years, 16-year-old students have come to us for a day. They get involved in laboratory experiments, talk to scientists and then take part in the discussion at a follow-on public event about some big health issue – 'Building Superhumans?' for example. It provokes thoughts, but crucially engagement like this supports youth voice in discussions about science and health. The students ask the questions and steer the discussion of a panel of invited celebrities and experts.

> *I now understand it is vital to be a part of the next generation to support the continuity of improving the population's general health and eliminating ailments threatening to life.*
>
> 16-year-old student after the 'Building Superhumans?' event

Adolescents are the new generation, the group who will hold the future in their hands. They'll form the next generation of voters, healthcare professionals, scientists and parents. So isn't it strange that most developed countries don't give adolescents the autonomy or responsibility that they feel that they deserve? As a highly innovative species, humans have always relied on the new ideas generated by each new generation to advance our societies and enhance our lives. However annoying or worrying it may be for older adults – especially their parents – the rebelliousness of adolescents has been a boon to us as a species.

What a Question

The 300-seat lecture theatre was packed for an evening public-engagement event around 'Building Superhumans?' Many young people were there. It was near the end of the evening and there was just time for one last question to the expert panel. A 16-year-old student stood up near the back, waiting nervously for the microphone to be passed to her.

'Do you think that everyone should be allowed to have a child?' she asked.

There was a gasp, then a ripple of embarrassed laughter, from the audience.

None of the panel – an Olympic medallist, a celebrity chef, a well-known TV scientist and the President of a medical Royal College – seemed immediately ready to answer the question. What was running through their minds? Was the question about the control of reproduction or the population explosion? Did the student have something particular in mind, maybe some personal experience which needed to be handled with extreme care? Did some members of the audience, parents and friends of the visiting students, think that the question was about eugenics – the ideas reminiscent of Nazi Germany and other fascist regimes that some potential parents were genetically 'inferior' and should not be allowed to have children?

But we knew what lay behind the question. The 16-year-old questioner was one of the students who had spent a day in our laboratories getting involved in some scientific research and being encouraged to think a little differently about what makes each of us who we are – the importance of the first 1,000 days in making a person.

The young woman asking the question had discovered by visiting us that these early days of life influence our futures. So her question was perhaps not so surprising. It demonstrated the vital importance she had attached to what she had learned that day – it had really surprised her – she may have wanted to shock the grown-ups into facing a new reality: just who has responsibility, anyway? She threw out a challenge to us, to take appropriate action. It was really a plea for information about what is needed to help every potential parent.

We wrote this book partly with this student in mind.

Get Our Act Together

As individuals we have a very powerful ability to act together. The use of social media and the local community action groups set up at short notice to meet the COVID-19 challenge across the world, really demonstrated this. They usually had no funding or established facilities and were assembled by like-minded people of all ages with no prior training. The impetus was the information widely disseminated about the threat of the virus to everyone.

Some politicians were fond of saying that we were all in the same boat in fighting the pandemic, to give the impression that everyone was being considered equally, until social media circulated the comment that we might all be in the same storm, but we were definitely not in the same boat. Some members of society were at greater risk, and so action groups were set up to protect them.

Public engagement, like the schemes and events we have run with young people, is recognised as an important part of building public understanding in many areas of science and a vital route for public opinion to be taken on board in the context of the science itself.

Every one of us, if equipped with understanding of the science of development, should be an important part of government attempts to 'follow the science' in policy-making.

The Buck Stops Here

In many instances the responsibility for giving the next generation a good start to life is placed firmly on the shoulders of parents. But we have seen that the effects of the environment on development may commence at conception, and so that environment has to be already established before conception. In fact, this places the responsibility with *prospective* parents – parents-to-be.

But responsibility is a slippery word, which often has negative implications. It is frequently used in what is called a 'retrospective' way, to hold someone or a group to account for events that have already taken place.

So do we cast the blame upon mothers, young women and adolescent girls, for the health problems which have their origins, in terms of risk, during our development? It's easy, but unfair and unhelpful. The quip 'A mother's place is … in the wrong' has a lot of truth in it.

What we really need is a sense of collective and 'prospective' responsibility – in other words the concept of working together to prevent something happening.

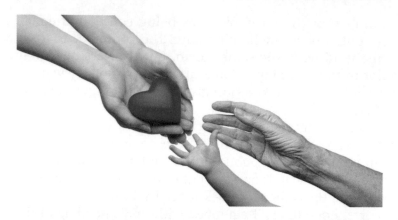

Figure 6.2 Developing healthy lives The call to action is to individuals, families and societies to make the gift of a healthier first 1,000 days to the next generation.
Green and Hanson, The Institute of Developmental Sciences, University of Southampton.

You may be the father of a child, or their grandfather. Or you may be too young to have even started thinking about having children. But you're still part of the cast of the play. In other words we, and this means not just parents but all of us, need to work together to ensure that as a society we give the next generation the best start to life. What do we, as the individuals who make up society, need to do?

This possibility of collective change does not necessarily have to be delegated to remote institutions like government or healthcare organisations, but can arise through all of us acting together.

Now it's up to all of us to decide how to use this straightforward new information about human development we've discussed, each in our own way

We can all do something about making development healthier, not only as individuals, but through families, groups of friends and society. Grandparents can contribute to supporting younger parents, a family or a school class could engage with a local food bank to make a healthier diet possible for disadvantaged couples and their children, a badminton club could raise funds to commission a YouTube video on the first 1,000 days for school students … we can all think of examples. Now it's up to all of us to decide how to use this straightforward new information about human development we've discussed, each in our own way.

We can all act to improve development.

The Gift

So it seems that we shouldn't put our trust in inherited genes just because our granny lived to be 99. Nor should we be lulled into a false sense of security by an uncle who ate a fried breakfast every morning and smoked into old age. Similarly, any 'lesson learned' from the premature death of a loved one is likely to be a complicated one.

We need to know about our early development. Parents, young people and, well, everyone really, might be forgiven for saying 'I had no idea. Why didn't anyone tell me about this?'

That's really why we wrote this book. We could have simply provided a list of things, based on current science, which young parents and potential parents, should do. And another one of things which they shouldn't do. But we decided not to do that.

There is plenty of advice to be had from highly qualified healthcare professionals on how to live a healthy life as adults. What this book does is to view our health from the point of view of our first 1,000 days. We hope that this stimulates new ideas as to why keeping healthy is so hard.

*Parents, young people, and, well, everyone real-
ly, might be forgiven for saying 'I had no idea.
Why didn't anyone tell me about this?'*

Perhaps the most important thing which we should all
remember is that, when it comes to giving the next generation the best possible start in life, fate does not come
into it.

The achievements of biomedical research over recent
decades have made it clear that, while genes are the tools
which our bodies use to develop, the plan of how we each
develop, and the use of the tools to do the job, is very
flexible. Over the first 1,000 days, the messages about life
which every person received from their parents set the
course of development.

Developmental differences are one of the reasons why
we are all unique, not only in how we look and behave,
but in how we will respond to the challenges of life which
we meet. New research in epigenetics has revealed some of
the underlying mechanisms involved.

It would indeed be very depressing if parents were told
soon after their baby was born, on the basis of the baby's
genetic makeup, how their child would turn out – how
they would cope with life, what diseases would probably
afflict them and perhaps what would be most likely to kill
them. Pre-implantation genetic diagnosis already tries to
do this with rare forms of genetic disease, which can give
helpful information under these specific conditions, but
imagine if this capability were extended to many other
aspects of life and future health including risk of later
NCDs.

So, is the 'call to action' we were seeking at the start of this
chapter to make sure that the planning of pregnancy is a priority? We don't just mean the idea of 'family planning' which
of course is an old-fashioned way of saying contraception or

abstinence. Of course, contraception is really important and there should be universal free access to it for anyone who wants it, worldwide.

But the planning goes much further than this.

The timing of pregnancy is very important. We have said that getting pregnant as a teenager is very often not the best option, either for the mother or her baby. The science shows that a mother who is herself still growing may not be able to support the growth and development of her fetus well. There is considerable evidence that being obese, having an unhealthy diet, smoking or taking recreational drugs can all send unhelpful messages to the embryo and fetus, and affect development.

It is important that sexually active men who may conceive a child are also aware that aspects of their lifestyle and unhealthy behaviours can affect the long-term health of their child. For many couples this new angle on gender equality may make life simpler.

Some of this evidence is rather non-specific – for example what is considered to be a 'healthy' diet is not very prescriptive. But this flexibility makes life easier in many ways. Other aspects are very specific, for example the need to take a folic acid supplement of 400 micrograms every day for a woman who may conceive.

What we are saying is that, whenever possible, couples should make a plan and prepare for pregnancy and parenthood.

Such planning will be much easier for them to do if they receive support, not just from family and friends but from society more widely. With colleagues, we have published articles in medical journals which argue strongly for greater emphasis in public health, education and social support for the preconception period.

We have explained that this should not just be directed at women, and it should not be allowed to be perpetuated as a gender issue, as if this is a priority for the entirety of a woman's reproductive life.

But it should mean that the ideas we have explored in this book are discussed in schools with children of all ages as appropriate.

It should mean as well that healthcare professionals of all types should see this as part of their jobs – not just primary healthcare providers and GPs but social workers, health visitors, pharmacists, dentists ... the list is extensive, but that should make it easier. Many GPs do not engage young people with this issue, not only for lack of time and information, but because they do not feel that it's necessary to open up a subject not widely appreciated as important.

Making those first 1,000 days as good as possible for our future children will give them the gift of healthy development and boundless opportunities for their future

---

Then of course we earnestly hope that governments of all persuasions will see the importance of improving our lives in our first 1,000 days. We are encouraged in this hope by the attention being given to it by policy-makers in some quarters, and by non-government agencies such as WHO or UNICEF. Making those first 1,000 days as good as possible for our future children will give them the gift of healthy development and boundless opportunities for their future.

There is one last point we want to stress.

In this book we have been considering the long-term effects of our first 1,000 days on our lives. But, when it comes to thinking about what we can do to give the next generation the best 1,000 day start to life, the timescale for action may be much shorter. In many ways, for every couple, the time period over which preparation is needed for the first 1,000 days of their child's life is quite short. It's likely to be three to six months before conception when societal and healthcare support needs to be in place.

We must think about what support they might need to make these preparations. This will help in persuading healthcare professionals and political decision-makers to provide it as they plan healthcare strategies for our future.

We hope that we have conveyed a story of optimism in this book. Development over our first 1,000 days is a time of amazing plasticity, when there is everything to play for in terms of helping a new person to have the best start to their life. All the experience of life of the parents, and of course of *their* parents, and those before … etc. stretching back perhaps over many generations, will have been filtered, assimilated and passed on in some form or other to this new generation.

This is a fantastic story of care, or of unconscious love we could say, communicated across inherited time.

Building on this optimism, there is much we can do as individuals, families and societies to make the gift of a healthier first 1,000 days to the next generation.

ACKNOWLEDGEMENTS

Between us, we have about 70 years of experience of researching the processes underlying early development, attending many hundreds of meetings from large international symposia to small workshops and engaging with a large number of colleagues from many disciplines and many countries. It is impossible to recognise the influences on our thinking which have come from these colleagues. We could not possibly acknowledge them all and we hope that they will forgive us for not singling out specific colleagues. We express our gratitude to them all.

We must however thank Dr Michael Penkler (Vienna) and Professor Carlos Blanco (Groningen) for their careful reading and comments on early versions of the manuscript. Giovanni Carrada (Rome) was enormously helpful in encouraging Mark to start writing the book, and his idea of 'the gift' which one generation passes to the next has been influential.

This book is not intended for the scientific or medical community, although we hope that they read it too. Over the years we have taught medical and science students and we are grateful to these past students for their influence on this book, whether through frank conversations or the energy they devoted to experiments, papers and presentations. Hopefully this book will be a resource to inspire the next generation of researchers or doctors to join this area of medical science and public health.

Over the years, we have tried to convey our passion for the science of human development to friends and families, attendees at science festivals, public talks or in schools. Whether they were bewildered or impressed by these conversations, we are indebted to them for provoking our thoughts and challenging the way we communicate this area of science. Clearly, few people are aware of the importance of the first 1,000 days of human development for lifelong health and we believe that this is a gaping hole in public health. In trying to raise awareness of this issue, this book should in many ways have been written years ago – but to do so required the input and steer from a wide range of people, and these conversations take time.

Jane Kitcher supported us and patiently produced drafts of sections of the book from notes and tapes. And, as ever, Donald Winchester from Watson Little Ltd has been a wise advisor and thoroughly supportive agent.

FURTHER READING

Bakermans-Kranenburg MJ, Lotz A, Alyousefi-van Dijk K, van IJzendoorn M. 'Birth of a Father: Fathering in the First 1,000 Days'. *Child Development Perspectives*. (2019) Dec;13(4):247–53.

Department for Health and Social Care, UK (2021) 'The best start for life: a vision for the 1001 critical days'. Online policy paper. www.gov.uk/government/publications/the-best-start-for-life-a-vision-for-the-1001-critical-days.

Gluckman P, Hanson M. (2008) *Mismatch: The Lifestyle Diseases Timebomb*. Oxford University Press.

Hanson MA and Gluckman PD. 'Early Developmental Conditioning of Later Health and Disease: Physiology or Pathophysiology?' *Physiological Reviews*. (2014) Oct;94(4):1027–76.

Karakochuk CD, Whitfield KC, Green TJ, Kraemer K, eds. (2017) *The Biology of the First 1,000 Days*. CRC Press.

McClure N. (2006) *The First 1000 Days: A Baby Journal*. Sasquatch Books.

Nathanielsz P. (2021) *Life Before Birth: The Challenges of Fetal Development*. 2nd ed. Life Course Health Press.

Thurow R. (2016) *The First 1000 Days: A Crucial Time for Mothers and Children – and the World*. PublicAffairs.

Woods-Townsend K, Hardy-Johnson P, Bagust L. 'A Cluster-Randomised Controlled Trial of the LifeLab Education Intervention to Improve Health Literacy in Adolescents'. *PLoS One*. (2021) May 5;16(5):e0250545.

INDEX